Push your Career Publish your Thesis

Science should be accessible to everybody. Share the knowledge, the ideas, and the passion about your research. Give your part of the infinite amount of scientific research possibilities a finite frame.

Publish your examination paper, diploma thesis, bachelor thesis, master thesis, dissertation, or habilitation treatises in form of a book.

A finite frame by infinite science.

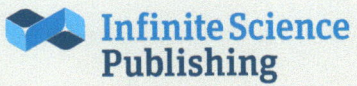

An Imprint of
Infinite Science GmbH
MFC 1 | Technikzentrum Lübeck
BioMedTec Wissenschaftscampus
Maria-Goeppert-Straße 1
23562 Lübeck
book@infinite-science.de
www.infinite-science.de

Editor

Thorsten M. Buzug
Institute of Medical Engineering
University of Lübeck
buzug@imt.uni-luebeck.de

Reihe: Medizinische Ingenieurwissenschaft und Biomedizintechnik

Diese Reihe umfasst Werke der Medizinischen Ingenieurwissenschaft und Biomedizintechnik, deren Themen strategisch unter den Zukunftstechnologien mit hohem Innovationspotenzial anzusiedeln sind. Als wesentliche Trends dieser Forschungsgebiete, sind die Schlüsselbereiche Computerisierung, Miniaturisierung und Molekularisierung zu nennen. Bei der Computerisierung sind dabei die inhaltlichen Schwerpunkte beispielsweise in der Bildgebung und Bildverarbeitung gegeben. Die Miniaturisierung spielt unter anderem bei intelligenten Implantaten, der minimalinvasiven Chirurgie aber auch bei der Entwicklung von neuen nanostrukturierten Materialien eine wichtige Rolle, und die Molekularisierung ist in der regenerativen Medizin aber auch im Rahmen der sogenannten molekularen Bildgebung ein entscheidender Aspekt. Forschungs- und Entwicklungspotenzial werden auch der Biophotonik und der minimal-invasiven Chirurgie unter Berücksichtigung der Robotik und Navigation zugeschrieben. Querschnittstechnologien wie die Mikrosystemtechnik, optische Technologien, Softwaresysteme und Wissenstechnologien sind dabei von hohem Interesse.

Maik Stille

Reconstruction of a 3-Dimensional Brain Volume from Fluorescent Images and its Co-Registration with Magnetic Resonance Imaging

Medical Engineering Science and Biomedical Engineering — Volume 9

Editor: Thorsten M. Buzug

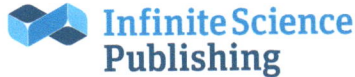

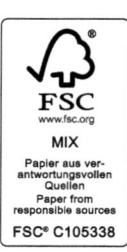

© 2015 Infinite Science Publishing
the BioMedTec Science Campus Publisher Lübeck

An Imprint of Infinite Science GmbH,
MFC 1 | BioMedTec Wissenschaftscampus
Maria-Goeppert-Straße 1
23562 Lübeck

Cover Design, Illustration: Uli Schmidts, metonym
Copy Editing: University of Lübeck, Institute of Medical Engineering

Publisher: Infinite Science GmbH, Lübeck, www.infinite-science.de
Print: Books on Demand GmbH, Norderstedt

ISBN Paperback: 978-3-945954-10-2

Das Werk, einschließlich seiner Teile, ist urheberrechtlich geschützt. Jede Verwertung ist ohne Zustimmung des Verlages und des Autors unzulässig. Dies gilt insbesondere für die elektronische oder sonstige Vervielfältigung, Bearbeitung, Übersetzung, Mikroverfilmung, Verbreitung und öffentliche Zugänglichmachung sowie die Einspeicherung und Verarbeitung in elektronischen Systemen.

Die Wiedergabe von Gebrauchsnamen, Handelsnamen, Warenbezeichnungen usw. in dieser Publikation berechtigt auch ohne besondere Kennzeichnung nicht zu der Annahme, dass solche Namen im Sinne der Warenzeichen- und Markenschutz-Gesetzgebung als frei zu betrachten wären und daher von jedermann verwendet werden dürften.

Bibliografische Information der Deutschen Nationalbibliothek:
Die Deutsche Nationalbibliothek verzeichnet diese Publikation in der Deutschen Nationalbibliografie; detaillierte bibliografische Daten sind im Internet über http://dnb.d-nb.de abrufbar.

Bibliographic information published by the Deutsche Nationalbibliothek
The Deutsche Nationalbibliothek lists this publication in the Deutsche Nationalbibliografie; detailed bibliographic data are available in the internet at http://dnb.d-nb.de.

Abstract

Background In the research of neuronal diseases, a comparison of magnetic resonance imaging (MRI) and histology sections is indispensable. While histology provides information about microscopic structures and chemical composition of brain tissue, in-vivo high-contrast MRI is a powerful tool for detecting pathologic structures in living animals. In clinic practice, the histology-MRI correspondence is often determined visually by experienced neuroscientists. This is a time-consuming and laborious procedure.

Methods The current thesis provides an imaging pipeline that automatically aligns histology sections to the anatomically corresponding position in the MRI. The imaging pipeline consists of a twofold approach that includes the reconstruction of a 3-dimensional brain volume from fluorescent images and its co-registration with MRI. For both steps an intensity based image registration algorithm is adapted. The transformation for the reconstruction is rigid, while the co-registration to the MRI volume is based on an initial rigid alignment that is subsequently refined by an affine registration step. In order to evaluate the proposed method, corresponding anatomical landmarks in MRI and histology were selected by experts.

Results The discrepancy after co-registration indicates an alignment error of $0.249\,\text{mm}$ for image data of healthy rat brains and $0.323\,\text{mm}$ for image data of animals that suffered a stroke. In due consideration of the resolution of the MRI with a voxel size of $0.234\,\text{mm} \times 0.234\,\text{mm} \times 0.600\,\text{mm}$ and a diagonal length of a given voxel of $0.685\,\text{mm}$ we obtain an accuracy that is below the resolution of the given image and by that acceptable for the present application.

Conclusion The accuracy achieved by the proposed reconstruction and registration pipeline enables a precise analysis of microstructural features seen in the histology sections and superimposed on the MRI. This in turn is extremely valuable for studying the cellular mechanisms that are responsible for signal changes in the MRI.

Contents

1 Introduction	1
2 Materials and Methods	7
2.1 Acquisition	7
2.2 Preprocessing	11
2.3 Reconstruction of Histology Volume	16
2.4 Co-Registration of Fluorescent Histology Images and MR Images	22
2.5 Validation Based on Landmarks	26
2.6 Registration Parameters	26
3 Results	31
3.1 Reconstruction of Histology Volume	31
3.2 Co-Registration of Fluorescent Histology Images and MR Images	32
4 Discussion	49
4.1 Source of Errors	50
4.2 Potential Improvements of the Imaging Pipeline	52
4.3 Future Work	53

5 Conclusion	55
Acknowledgement	57
Abbreviations	59
References	61

1
Introduction

Small animals like rats, mice, rabbits, or monkeys are widely used to improve the understanding of complex pathophysiological processes underlying diseases of the central nervous system [1 and 2]. Along the investigation of degenerative diseases like Alzheimer's or Parkinson's, neuroscientists of the Institute of Psychiatry, King's College London study animals that have suffered a stroke. According to the world health organization, stroke is the second leading cause of death world wide and the number one reason for disability in the United States and Europe[1].

Investigations of progression of cerebral ischaemia in small animal models include monitoring effects of therapeutic agents and obtaining signal changes in in-vivo magnetic resonance imaging (MRI). In addition, a direct correlation between post mortem histology and MRI is needed for validation of cell tracking studies [3] and in-vivo molecular imaging. The combination of information gained from different imaging modalities increases the diagnosis accuracy and lead to a comprehensive understanding of anatomical and pathophysiological structures. In conjunction with histology the cellular mechanisms responsible for signal changes in MRI can be studied precisely.

The data of imaging modalities like MRI and histology are highly incongruent and unprofitable for comparison. Image properties like field of view, dimensions, resolution, or contrast are inherently different due to the characteristics of MRI and histology images. In addition, differences in the accusation of slices in the two imaging modalities are observable. While the slice sampling in MRI is contiguous, the sampling in histology is sparse. In order to bring both image modalities in the same space, a mathematical method named multimodal image registration is required,

---

[1] http://www.who.int/mediacentre/factsheets/fs310/en/index.html

which determines a coordinate mapping between the two modalities [4–6]. This procedure is highly complicated by distortions that occur in brain tissue during the extraction, fixation, and staining process. Distortions may include shrinkage, bending, stretching, or folds of tissue with respect to the MR images.

Furthermore, a direct 2-dimensional alignment of histology sections to MRI slices is in most of the cases unfavourable. In general it cannot be ensured that histology sections are cut in the same angle as slices are acquired during MRI scanning [7]. A further complicating factor is that histology and MRI slices normally do not have the same thickness and slice-sampling. In order to avoid these problems, an initial 3-dimensional reconstruction of the histology volume is desirable, followed by a 3-dimensional co-registration of the histology and MRI volume.

A few articles that discuss the reconstruction of brain sections can be found throughout literature [8–10]. Here, every pair of consecutive images in the stack is registered to recover their geometrical coherent 3-dimensional alignment. The registration process is complicated by the fact that image pairs are not of the same but of similar objects. Beare et al. [11] gave 2008 an overview of five different methods to align microscope images of Nissl-stained sections of mouse brain to form a 3-dimensional image volume. The automated image registration methods include the use of fiducial markers. Drill holes were used for quality measurement and as a cue for registration. Obviously this leads to destruction of brain tissue and is therefore undesirable.

Another approach to reconstruct a histology volume is performed under the use of a so-called blockface [12–14]. Here, the tissue block is fixed in a special frame and digitally photographed prior the cutting of each section. The method takes advantage of the fact the position of the brain stays the same during the sectioning and the reconstruction of the blockface volume can be performed by simply stacking up the digital images. The stained histology volume can be reconstructed by registering the tissue sections to the blockface images. Choe et al. (2011) presented a blockface method to combine light microscopic images with a ex-vivo MRI volume of an owl monkey brain [15]. After manually segmentation of the blockface images, a 2-dimensional slice- to-slice registration of the microscopic images with the blockface images is performed. Finally, the MRI volume is 3-dimensional registered with the reconstructed blockface volume. The approach showed an accuracy of 0.324 mm but suffers a disadvantage in competing with other methods since the costs for the additional purchase of a blockface frame is relatively high.

An early alternative is a landmark based co-registration [16–19]. Li et al. [18], for example, presented a co-registration of MRI and histology for cerebral ischaemia in small animal models. After manually identifying corresponding slices between the two imaging modalities, a guide-line-assisted manual selection of landmarks was performed. A thin plate spline transformation was then used to align corresponding images [18]. A more automated approach was presented by Jacobs et al. [17]. They used a head and hat surface based registration algorithm [20] where landmark points were automatically sampled along the image contours. However, although surface contours can be almost perfectly registered, it is not guaranteed that internal structures of the brain are also accurately aligned. Especially if distortions occur during sectioning. In [19] a method based on two types of automatically identified landmarks for images of prostate is presented. Landmarks are not only located on the prostate boundaries but also on salient internal anatomical regions. Unfortunately, the method for the selection of internal landmarks is extremely influenced by the anatomy of the structure investigated and the quality of the acquired image data. The approach showed a mean error of 0.820 mm compared to manually selected landmarks.

Xiao et al. presented recently a method for histology and MR images of prostate where initially a slice-to-slice correspondence is assumed [21]. After group-wise comparison of mutual information between MRI and histology slices, a pseudo histology volume was created by filling the gap between slices with zero-value slices. In order to compensate the fact that the orientation of the 2-dimensional histology slices and the axial MRI slices may not be identical, a 3-dimensional co-registration of the histology and MRI volume is performed.

With the goal of building an atlas of the human basal ganglia, Ourselin et al. (2001) presented a method that adapted an intensity based registration approach [22]. The main idea of the presented algorithm is to divide images into blocks. Only the best corresponding block is then used for registration in order to reduce the influence of distortion in histology sections. The authors suggested a rigid transformation for the reconstruction of the histology volume and the correlation coefficient as a similarity measure. For the co-registration with MRI the same block-matching strategy is adapted. Here, an initial rigid registration is followed by an affine registration while correlation ratio is used as a similarity measure. Since the algorithm uses only local information, namely the area of one block, for the registration it may not align anatomical features of interest outside this block accurately. As a consequence the proposed method suffers from a misalignment of the corpus callosum after co-registration [22].

The object of the current article is to design a simple and accurate imaging pipeline for the co-registration of in-vivo MRI of a rat brain with corresponding ex-vivo fluorescent histology sections. The superimposition of histology section on MRI will allow a detailed investigation of microstructural features seen in the histology and superimposed on the MRI as well as the study of the source of intensity variances in the in-vivo MRI volume. The proposed pipeline consists of a twofold approach that can be divided into the reconstruction of the 3-dimensional brain volume from fluorescent histology images and its co-registration with the MRI volume. Both steps are performed using an intensity based approach. The reconstruction of the histology volume is made up of a number of 2-dimensional registrations of consecutive slices. The transformation chosen for these registration steps only allows rotation and translation in order to preserve the shape of the tissue. The sum of squared distances is used as similarity measure in order to to drive the registration. Following from the 3-dimensional reconstruction of the fluorescent histology volume, a matching of histology slices to non-axial MRI slices is possible. The final co-registration of the reconstructed histology volume and the MRI volume leads to a geometrically correct histology volume. Here, the resultant transformation of an initial rigid registration is used as a starting point for an affine registration. Normalised mutual information is adopted as a distance measure. After spatial alignment, a direct correspondence of the two image modalities is enabled.

There has been a lack of a convincing evaluation in the literature to date [7 and 21–24]. The illustration of superimposed histology on MR images is only advantageous for experts. For a non-professional, an evaluation based on visual inspection is hard, especially if different imaging modalities are involved. Another disadvantage of this evaluation method is the absence of quantification, which makes it difficult to determine a gradual improvement and an objective assessment between techniques. On the other hand, a validation based on the evaluation of a similarity or distance measurement gives an indication of the quality of the registration but provides little information about the match of anatomy. An analysis of the overlap of two volumes by utilising a region-based quality metric [25–27] or model-based evaluation [28] gives information about correspondence of the surface but suffers from a detailed evaluation of the inner structure–unless an extensive masking and labelling of anatomical features has been performed.

Another way to investigate the alignment of the two imaging modalities is by using anatomical landmarks. Selecting corresponding landmarks in MRI and histology before co-registration has the advantage that a detailed description of mismatch can be given by summing up the distance between anatomical landmarks after co-registration. Ideally, the previously selected points possess the same position after the proposed imaging pipeline is applied.

In chapter 2 the analysis pipelines for histology reconstruction and histology to MRI registration are described in detail. An evaluation of the co-registration based on anatomical landmarks for normal and abnormal brain images can be found in chapter 3. In chapter 4 technical and methodological issues, as well as how the application challenges were solved, are discussed. A brief conclusion is drawn in chapter 5.

2

Materials and Methods

Here, a pipeline for the 3-dimensional reconstruction of fluorescent histology image data and its co-registration with the corresponding MRI volume is presented. The pipeline, which is illustrated in figure 2.1, is structured as follows. In-vivo magnetic resonance imaging (MRI) was performed for animals that are part of a study of stroke using a rat model. After euthanasia, the animals were prepared for immunohistochemistry and the histology images were acquired. Following preprocessing of the histology and MR image data, a 3-dimensional reconstruction of the histology volume is performed. In section 2.4 the co-registration of MRI and fluorescent histology is described. Finally, validation methods are presented that are used in order to perform an evaluation and quality control of the proposed imaging pipeline. A detailed overview of the used techniques can be found in the following sections. The proposed imaging pipeline is developed under heavy use of the open source image registration toolkit elastix [29]. A summary of the experimentally determined registration parameters is given in section 2.6.

2.1 Acquisition

The presented imaging pipeline was tested and validated on MRI and histology images acquired as part of a study of stroke. In the following sections details of the used rat model and the acquisition of the image data is given.

2.1.1 Animals

For the acquisition of the fluorescent histology and MRI volumes Sprague Dawley rats (Harlan, UK) were used. Rats were acclimatised for at least a week prior to

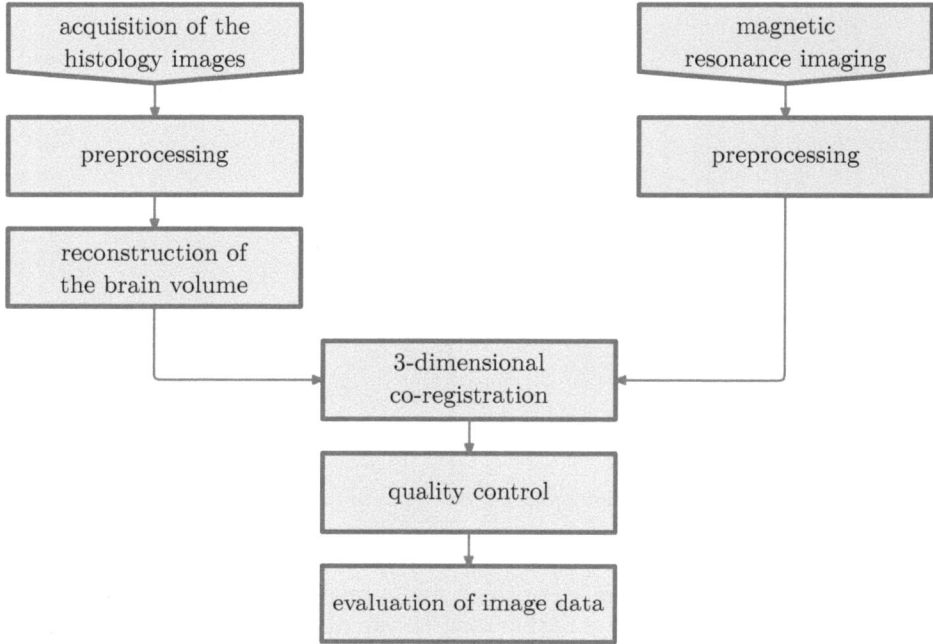

Figure 2.1 Overview of the image-processing pipeline.

surgery to create the disease model. All procedures were in accordance with the UK Animals (Scientific) Procedures Act 1986 and the ethical review process of King's College London. Animals were on a 12 h light:12 h dark schedule with food and water available ad lib.

2.1.2 Middle Cerebral Artery Occlusion

In order to study the pathophysiology of stroke, a model for cerebral ischaemia is used. Middle cerebral artery occlusion (MCAO) is the most commonly used method for cerebral ischaemic stroke in rats since it represents the most prevalent form of stroke in humans [30].

Animals between 280-330 g were either allocated for sham or 60 minutes of right transient MCAOsurgery [31]. Briefly, animals were anaesthetised with isoflourane (4% induction, 2% maintenance) in a mixture of O_2 and medical air (50:50). Temporary ligatures were placed on the ipsilateral external and common carotid to stop the flow of blood to the internal carotid artery. The tip of the thread was advanced 18-20 mm from the cervical carotid bifurcation or until reaching resistance from the ostium of the middle cerebral artery in the circle of Willis. Following occlusion, animals were tested for spontaneous circling and forelimb flexion [31]. Occluded animals were re-anaesthetised and the thread was removed. Neurological scoring and post-operative care were given daily until animals recovered pre-operative weight.

2.1.3 Magnetic Resonance Imaging

^{1}H MRI was performed using a horizontal bore 7 T MRI scanner. For the duration of the scanning session the animals were anaesthetised with isoflourane (4% induction, 2% maintenance) in a mixture of O_2:N_2O (30:70). The magnetic resonance imaging (MRI) consisted of a fast spin echo sequence with an echo time T_E of 60 ms. 45 slices with a thickness of 0.6 mm were collected at an in-plane resolution of 0.234 mm per pixel edge length. Since the field of view of the scanner amounts to 3 cm × 3 cm the digitised images consists of a 128 × 128 matrix for each of the 45 slices. Passive shimming was performed in order to align the gradients in the magnet such that the data acquired is homogenous.

2.1.4 Histological Assessments

After final MRI scanning the animals were given a lethal dose of sodium pentobarbitol (60 mg/kg i.p.) followed by intracardial perfusion of first 0.9% NaCl and then 4% ice-cold paraformaldehyde in 0.2 M phosphate buffered saline (PBS). The dissected brains were rinsed in cryoprotective solution (30% sucrose in PBS) for at least 24 h before they were cut on a cryostat (Microm Cryo-Star HM 560) at -24 °C into 50 μm thick coronal sections. The tissue was stored frozen at -20 °C before used for immunohistochemistry.

2.1.5 Immunohistochemistry

Hydrophobic barriers were drawn around pre-mounted tissue using a wax pen (Dako Ltd, Denmark) on coverslips to allow immunohistochemical staining directly onto slides. Primary antibodies were added at appropriate dilution after blocking of endogenous background staining (10% normal rabbit serum, 0.1% Triton X-100 in PBS 1 hr). Incubations with primary antibodies were performed overnight in fresh blocking solution at 4 °C and made visible using fluorescence-conjugated secondary antibodies in PBS for 2 hours at room temperature.

Different stains were applied to different adjacent sections depending on the experiments they were involved in. However, all sections were stained with the fluorescent stain DAPI (4',6-diamidino-2-phenylindole) that can pass through the membrane of

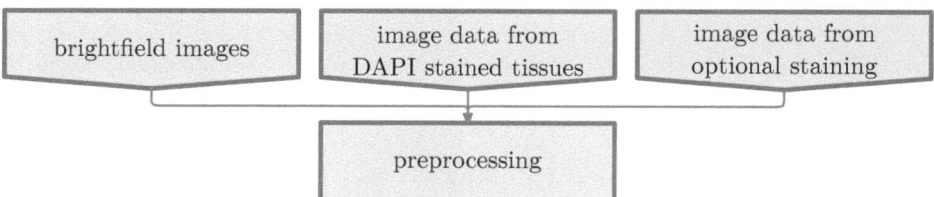

Figure 2.2 Acquisition of the histology images. Beside the collection of image data from DAPI stained tissue images from other optional stains were acquired. Bright field images were collected within the same space as the fluorescent images and can therefor easily be used for masking as described in section 2.2.1.

a cell. Out of the complete sequence of slices for one animal only every tenth slice was available for processing, which makes an overall amount of 21 to 24 slices per extracted brain. Sections used for processing were additionally stained with GFAP (Glial Fibrillary Acidic Protein) in order to study glia scar formation.

2.1.6 Microscopy and Digitisation

Under the use of a fluorescence microscope, images were collected from 9 animals–6 animals of a control group and 3 animals with a stroke (see section 2.1.2). Fluorescence microscopy is a special method of optical microscopy and is used to study properties of organic or inorganic substances. A fluorescence microscope is based on the physical principle of phosphorescence and florescence where so called fluorophores are illuminated by a light with a specific wavelength. Due to the absorption of light the fluorophores re-emit energy of a different, longer, wavelength that can be detected through a microscope objective. The use of a special filter in the microscope ensures that the distribution of a single fluorophore is imaged at a time.

When bounded to double-stranded DNA DAPI has a maximum absorption wavelength of 358 nm (ultraviolet) and re-emits a maximum emission of 461 nm (blue).

Fluorescence histology images were obtained on a Zeiss Stereo Lumar V12 with excitation by fluorescence light source and collection by a Zeiss AxioCam HRc. The digitisation result in images with a resolution of (1388 px × 1040 px) while a magnification of 16 was used. Considering the field of view of the microscope this implies that the size of a pixel in the digitised images corresponds to an area of 11.97 μm × 11.97 μm . The high resolution of the fluorescent histology images allow a detailed observation of anatomical structures as the hippocampus, the thalamus, or the corpus callosum. Figure 2.3 shows examples of collected fluorescent histology images.

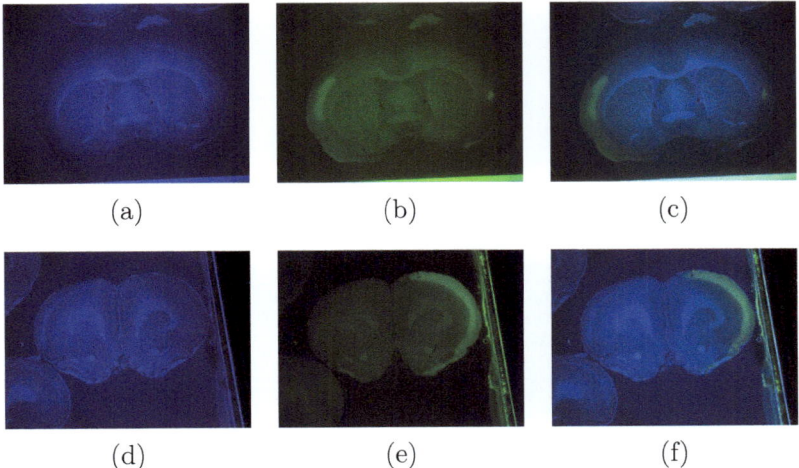

Figure 2.3 Collected fluorescent image data. (a) and (d) image data of DAPI stained tissue, (b) and (e) image data of GFAP[2] stained tissue. Image (c) and (d) shows the overlay of the two different stains.

Beside the acquisition of image data from DAPI stained tissue bright field images were collected (figure 2.2). In bright field microscopy the sample is illuminated with white light from below and observed from above. The contrast in the images is caused by absorbance of light in dense areas of the sample. Due to a better signal to noise ratio these images are used for masking as described in section 2.2.1. The collection of bright field images can be performed with the same microscope used to acquire the fluorescence images.

2.2 Preprocessing

In order to perform the 3-dimensional reconstruction of the histology volume and the following co-registration with the MRI volume, several preprocessing steps need

---

[2] GFAP (Glial Fibrillary Acidic Protein) is used to detect glia cells, which provide support and electrical isolation for neurones.

to be applied to the histology image data (section 2.2.1) and the MRI volume (section 2.2.2).

2.2.1 Histology Images

The necessary preprocessing steps that are performed before using the histology image data to reconstruct the 3-dimensional volume are presented in figure 2.4.

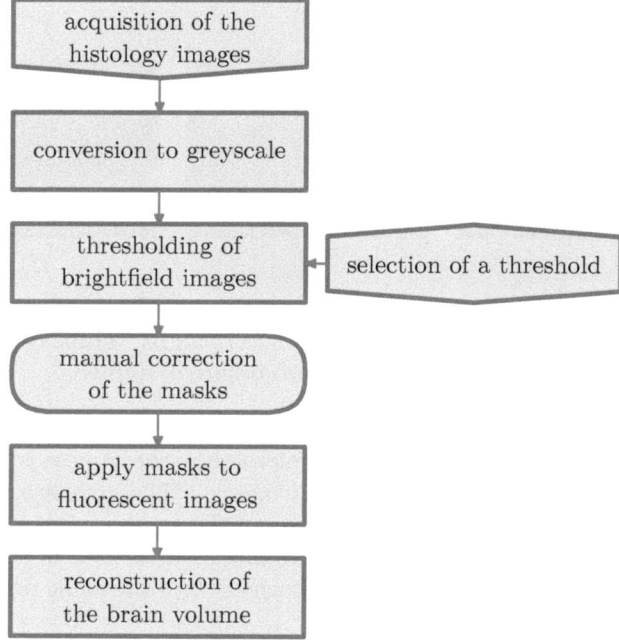

Figure 2.4 Pipeline for the preprocessing of the histology images. After converting the image data into a greyscale representation, a masking technique is applied,.

Since the imaging pipeline and consequently the registration techniques work on grey level intensities, the data needs to be available in a greyscale representation. Note that, due to the use of colour filters while collecting histology image data only a specific frequency is used in order to acquire the images. Generally, images are represented in a pseudo colouring, with colours matching the wavelength of the acquired fluorescent light, when received from the microscope software. In order to convert the data back into greyscale representation, a single channel was extracted from the pseudo-coloured images. For instance, the image data of DAPI stained tissue is converted by extracting the blue channel of the RGB representation.

Since all image data is represented by grey values we now can define a d-dimensional image I as a mapping that assigns every spatial point x belonging to a certain set $\Omega \subset \mathbb{R}^d$ a grey value $I(x)$ with $d \in \mathbb{N}$ so that $I : \Omega \to \mathbb{R}$.

As illustrated in figure 2.3 the collected histology image data suffers from a substantial amount of structure in the background. Due to the limitation of space on the slide it is rarely the case that only a single section occurs in the image. Generally different parts of tissue can be found that occasionally overlie or touch. In images of tissue sections that are located on the edge of a glass slide it is most likely that the border appears and structure beyond the slide occurs.

It is essential for the reconstruction and the co-registration that the images are reduced to the tissue of a single section. Therefor a masking technique is developed that allows the extraction of the object from the background.

A segmentation method that is based on a simple threshold was not feasible for the fluorescent histology image data. The emission of light by the fluorescent tissue has the disadvantage that the junction from tissue to background is not characterised by an acceptable contrast (figure 2.5). Emitted light does not only reflect in the direction of the excitatory light but in all various angles, which leads to a visible glow of the tissue. Matters were complicated further by the fact that the staining fades out over time and introduced a weaker signal near the edges of the tissue, which causes a poor contrast between object and background. The situation is exemplarily illustrated in figure 2.5.

Despite the lack of a sufficient contrast between object and background, masking was performed under the use of bright field images. The bright field images are characterised by a excellent signal to noise ratio. As illustrated in figure 2.5 one can recognise an abrupt change in the grey values on the border of object and background. On basis of the significant decrease of the grey values outside the object the images were normalised such that the background is zero and the foreground is greater than zero. This was performed by using a threshold technique. A threshold $\tau_i \in [0, 255]$ is selected by the user for each image I_i such that

$$i(x) \geq \tau_i \text{ if } x \in \Theta_i$$
$$\text{and } i(x) < \tau_i \text{ if } x \notin \Theta_i$$

where $\Theta_i \subseteq \Omega_i$ denotes the set of non background pixel, $\Omega_i \subset \mathbb{R}^2$ denotes the spatial domain of the image I_i and $x \in \Omega_i$.

Theoretically each image would require a individual threshold τ_i. However, in our experiments the same value $\tilde{\tau} = 11$ has proven to be sufficient for all i.

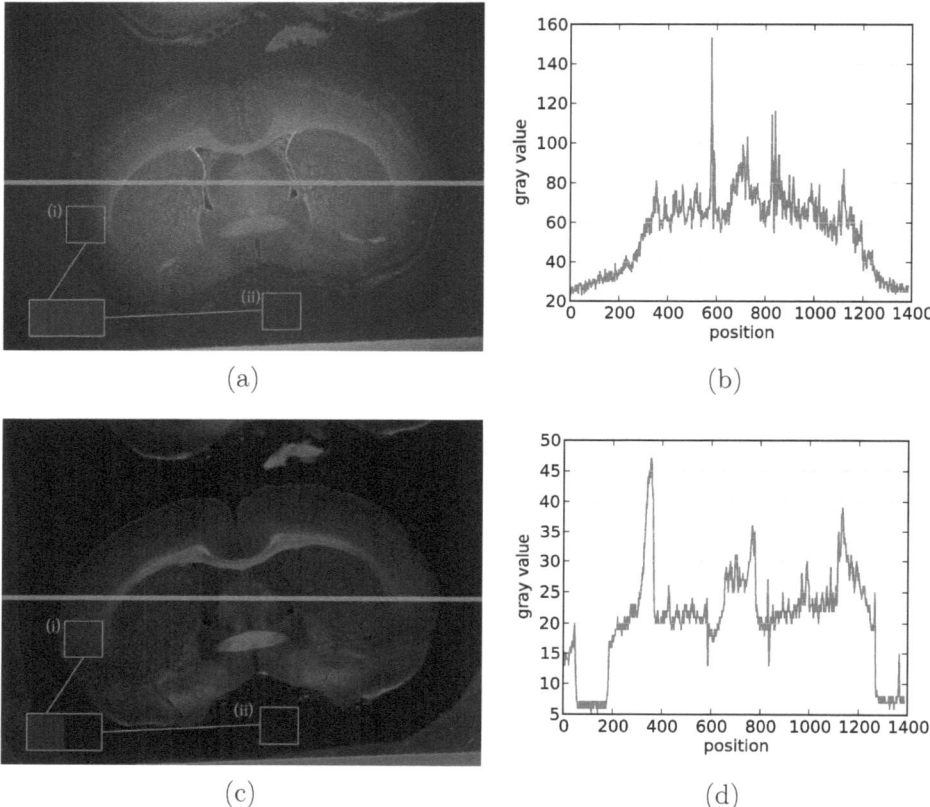

Figure 2.5 Comparison of a fluorescent histology image with a bright field image. The fluorescent image (a) is not qualified for masking as it shows a poor grey value contrast between the object and the background (box (i) and (ii)). The grey value profile along the red line in (a) signalised a soft junction from tissue to background as illustrated in (b). In comparison the signal to noise ratio in the bright field image of the same section (c) is more promising. The diagram in (d) indicates a significant change in the grey values along the border of the tissue. A thresholding technique with a threshold $\tilde{\tau} = 11$ can be applied.

After applying the threshold $\tilde{\tau}$ to all images $I_i \in S_a$, where S_a denotes the image stack of histology images for an animal a, we get a binary mask M_i for each image I_i. In order to remove noise and tiny structures in the mask the morphologic operations

Preprocessing 15

erosion and dilation (also known as opening) were performed as described in [32]. The amount of iterations of the dilation process can be used as a parameter to adjust the size of the mask. Therefore one can control how much of the structure surrounding the tissue will be included in the resulting image. This can be practical for the registration process since the border of the object (tissue) is taken into account as a feature of the image. All remaining holes were eliminated by applying region-filling. Since the mask still contains regions of different tissue sections and undesired structures of the glass slide (e.g. the edge of the slide as illustrated in figure 2.3), these areas need to be removed. This is done manually by the user.

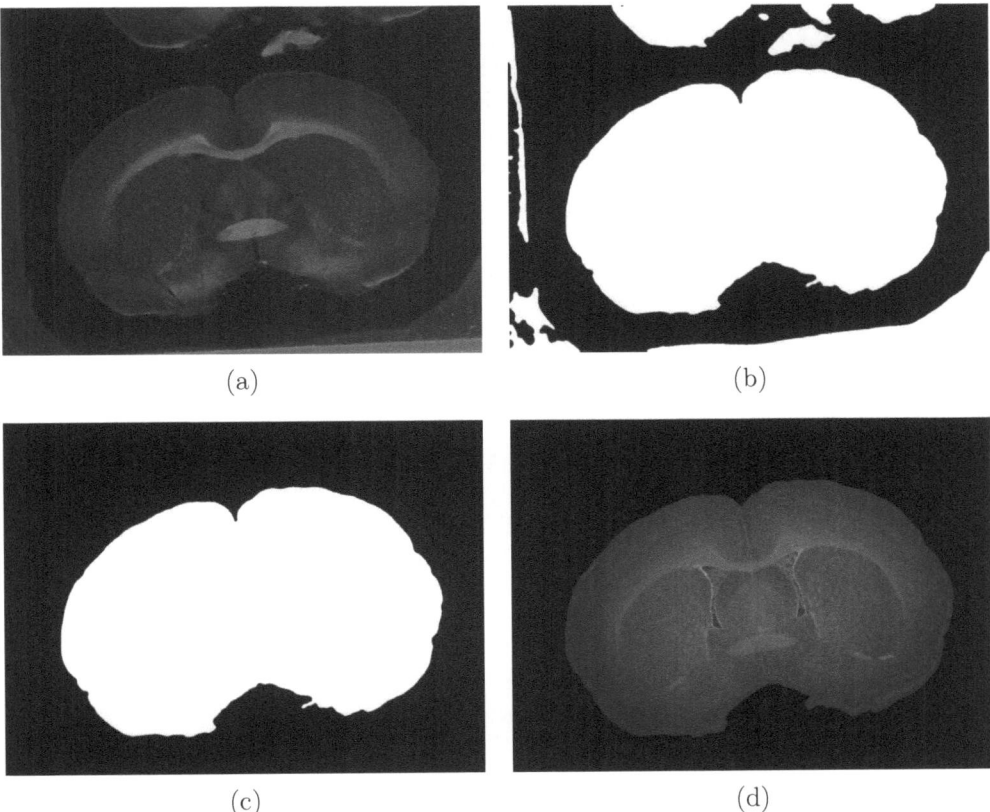

Figure 2.6 In this figure the process of the masking is illustrated. Image (a) shows the bright field image after grey scale conversion. (b) shows the mask after thresholding, opening, and region filling. After manual correction (c), the mask can be applied to the fluorescence image (d).

The resulting mask is now used to extract the tissue of the fluorescent images from the background. Hereby, every pixel that does not coincide with the mask is set to the background colour 0. This approach delivers satisfying segmentation results after testing it with three different stacks of histology images S_a where $a \in [1,3]$. An example for the masking pipeline is illustrated in figure 2.6.

2.2.2 Magnetic Resonance Images

After in-vivo scanning, neuroscientists of the Institute of Psychiatry, King's College London extracted the brains of 9 animals from full head MRI volumes. In order to reduce the amount of background voxel and therefore the amount of voxel used for the processing, cropping was applied. The desired shape was calculated by determining the minimum and maximum index of object voxel in all three directions. The dimensions of the volume after cropping differ from 61 to 64 voxel in x-direction, 42 to 48 voxel in y-direction, and 21 to 24 voxel in z-direction.

Since the MRI volume and the reconstructed histology volume (see section 2.3) need to have the same dimensions for the registration, the cropped MRI volume was up-sampled on the basis of a nearest-neighbour method. An up-sampling with a factor of 10 for the x- and y-direction was performed with success. The number of slices (z-direction) were left untouched. Note that the resulting MRI slices have a resolution of approximately $620\,\text{px} \times 440\,\text{px}$ with a field of view of $3\,\text{cm} \times 3\,\text{cm}$.

2.3 Reconstruction of Histology Volume

In order to perform a 3-dimensional co-registration of the MRI volume and fluorescent histology image data a reconstruction of the histology volume is required. The shape of the histology volume is based on the position of tissue in the image data. Adjacent slices are misaligned but show similar appearance. The main idea is to realign the section by maximising the agreement in appearance to correct the misalignment and therefore the shape of the volume. This depends highly on the in-plane anatomy, which is changing slowly in the slice direction compared to the distance between sections.

The process of finding a suitable spatial transformation for an image so that it best matches–becomes more similar to–a reference image is called image registration [4–6]. This process requires a mathematical formalisation for the similarity of two images. One way to do this is by defining a distance measure or cost-function $\mathcal{D}: \mathbb{R}^{2d} \to \mathbb{R}$, which is modulated such that $\mathcal{D}(I_1, I_2) < \mathcal{D}(I_1, I_3)$ if image I_1 and I_2 are more similar to each other than I_1 and I_3.

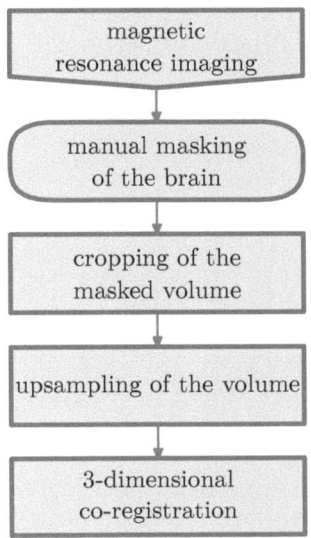

Figure 2.7 Pipeline for the preprocessing of the magnetic resonance images. Before using the MRI volume for the co-registration the brain is manually extracted from the skull and the volume is cropped to the size of the remaining tissue. Because of the poor resolution of the MRI volume up-sampling was performed.

A mathematical description of the registration problem can now be written as follows. Given a reference image R, a template image T, and a distance measure $\mathcal{D}: \mathbb{R}^{2d} \to \mathbb{R}$ find a transformation $\varphi: \mathbb{R}^d \to \mathbb{R}^d$ such that

$$\mathcal{D}(R, T \circ \varphi) = min. \tag{2.1}$$

2.3.1 Initial Alignment

Before the 2-dimensional registration of reference image R and template image T is applied a basic initial alignment is performed by utilising the centre of mass of both images. In general the centre of mass P_{COM} is defined as

$$P_{COM} = \frac{\int \rho(r) r \, dr}{\int \rho(r) \, dr} \tag{2.2}$$

with the mass density ρ and a position r. If we apply this to an image I and interpret the grey values as a density distribution P_{COM} can be written as

$$P_{COM}(I) = \frac{\sum_{x \in \Omega} I(x) x}{\sum_{x \in \Omega} I(x)} \qquad (2.3)$$

with $x \in \Omega \subset \mathbb{R}^2$.

Based on this a distance vector $t = P_{COM}(R) - P_{COM}(T)$ is calculated and the target image T is translated with the transformation $\varphi_t(x) = x + t$ thereby aligning the centres of mass of the two images.

2.3.2 Rigid Transformation

In order to solve the registration problem described in formula 2.1 a transformation needs to be defined with respect to the requirements of the reconstruction of the volume.

Since it is desirable to preserve the structure and shape of the sections a rigid transformation, which only allows rotation and translation is used to align the images. The rigid transformation is defined by

$$\varphi(x) = Qx + b \qquad (2.4)$$

where $Q \in \mathbb{R}^{d \times d}$ is orthogonal with $\det Q = 1$ and $b = \mathbb{R}^d$.

2.3.3 Sum of Squared Differences

For monomodal image registration problems it is common to use a intensity based approach that minimises the so-called sum of squared differences (SSD) [23 and 33]. The SSD similarity measure is based on the assumption that corresponding areas in two images are assigned identical grey values. Mathematically defined is the SSD distance measure $\mathcal{D}^{SSD}: \mathbb{R}^{2d} \to \mathbb{R}$ by

$$\mathcal{D}^{SSD}[R,T] := \frac{1}{2}\|T - R\|_{L_2}^2 = \frac{1}{2}\int_{\mathbb{R}^d} (T(x) - R(x))^2 \, dx. \qquad (2.5)$$

2.3.4 Adaptive Stochastic Gradient Descent Optimisation

In order to find an optimal alignment of two images R and T it is necessary to find the right parameters p of the transformation φ_p such that the distance measure

$\mathcal{D}(R, T \circ \varphi_p)$ yields ideally a global minimum. This leads to an optimisation problem, which is solved by an optimiser. A gradient based optimiser works by iteratively changing the parameters p of the transformation φ_p by using the gradient of a distance measure $\mathcal{D}$ until the optimum is reached. In the proposed imaging pipeline, the adaptive stochastic gradient descent optimisation (ASGD) for image registration introduced by Klein et al. [34] is used. The advantage of this method compared to naive optimiser is a stochastic estimation of the similarity measure $\mathcal{D}$. The method, which is based on the theoretical work by Plakhov and Cruz [35], reduces the computational cost per iteration by using an approximation $\tilde{g}$ of the true derivate $g = \partial \mathcal{D}/\partial p$ at p_k. The approximation $\tilde{g}$ is computed using a subset of pixels instead of all pixels. Therefore the approximated gradient $\tilde{g}$ is defined as

$$\tilde{g} = g + \epsilon \qquad (2.6)$$

where ϵ denotes the approximation error. The iterative scheme of the optimisation method is mathematically described by

$$p_{k+1} = p_k - \delta(t_k)\tilde{g}_k \quad \text{with } k = 0, 1, ..., K \qquad (2.7)$$

with

$$\delta(t) = \frac{a}{(t+A)} \quad \text{with } a > 0 \text{ and } A \geq 1 \qquad (2.8)$$

and with

$$t_{k+1} = max\{t_k + f(-\tilde{g}_k^T \tilde{g}_{k-1}),\ 0\}, \qquad (2.9)$$

where f denotes a sigmoid function and a, A, t_0, t_1, and the initial transformation parameters p_0 are user-defined arguments. The step-size δ is evaluated at the time t that is adapted depending on the inner product of the approximated gradient $\tilde{g}_k$ and the previous gradient $\tilde{g}_{k-1}$. This leads to a larger step size if the gradients in two consecutive iterations point in the same direction and a reduced step size otherwise. This optimisation approach has shown to be suitable for the proposed registration problem.

2.3.5 Multi-resolution

As suggested in the literature before [23] a multi-resolution approach is used. This strategy takes advantage of a pyramid of different data complexity to increase the chance of a successful registration. In the proposed 2-dimensional registration the pyramid is based on three resolutions where each layer is smoothed with a Gaussian filter of a different standard deviation ($\sigma = 4.0, 2.0, 1.0$ pixel). The result of layer l is used as an initial transformation for the registration at layer $l+1$.

2.3.6 Order of Registration

The reconstruction of the histology volume is performed by solving 20 to 22 optimisation problems per animal. In this context, the order of the 2-dimensional registration is a crucial factor and highly affects the result of the reconstruction. Therefore, a definition of the registration order was required that gives good results and can be applied consistently across different data sets. A method that has shown to be practicable, is by defining a reference image $I_{i_{fix}} \in S_a$ that represents a fix point in the image stack S_a. For simplification, image $I_{i_{fix}}$ will be written as I_{fix}. All other images $I_i \in S_a \setminus \{I_{fix}\}$ are registered with respect to the fixed image I_{fix}. Obviously, slice I_{fix} is not transformed at all. It is possible to choose the reference image automatically. For instance, by selecting the image with the maximum number of non zero pixels [23] or by choosing the slice index in the middle $i_{fix} = |S_a|/2$. However, the proposed method gives the option to define the fix point manually in order to avoid a reference image with artefacts that could affect the registration.

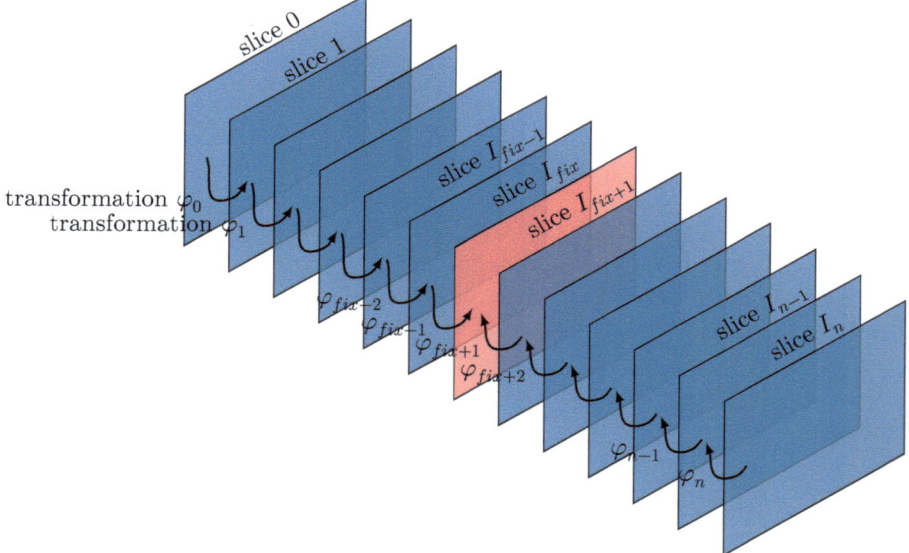

Figure 2.8 Order for the 2-dimensional registration of fluorescent histology slices. Slice $I_{fix} \in S_a$ denotes a fix point of the image stack S_a. All images $I \in S_a \setminus \{I_{fix}\}$ are registered with respect to I_{fix}.

After choosing a reference image I_{fix} all images $I \in S_a \setminus \{I_{fix}\}$ are registered to its neighbour $I_j \in S_a$ that is the nearest to the fixed image (figure 2.8). Consequently is $j = i + 1$ if $i < i_{fix}$ and $j = i - 1$ if $i > i_{fix}$. The overall transformation $\hat{\varphi}_i$ for an image $I_i \in S_a \setminus \{I_{fix}\}$ is due to the concatenation of transformations φ_i that result from the individual registrations.

$$\hat{\varphi}_i = \varphi_i \times \varphi_{i+1} \times \ldots \times \varphi_{fix-2} \times \varphi_{fix-1} \qquad (2.10)$$

where $i < i_{fix}$. Analogously, the overall transformation $\hat{\varphi}_i$ with $i > i_{fix}$ is defined by

$$\hat{\varphi}_i = \varphi_i \times \varphi_{i-1} \times \ldots \times \varphi_{fix+2} \times \varphi_{fix+1}. \qquad (2.11)$$

In order do build a volume the transformed image stack $\hat{S}_a$ were converted into a NIfTI-file[3] and all necessary parameter were set (e.g. dimension of pixel, xyz unit).

It is not to be expected to get a spatial correct shape of the histology volume since information for the reconstruction of the 3-dimensional volume are only available in the through-plane direction and therefore ambiguous. In figure 2.9 this problem is illustrated while considering a binary volume. Using grey value sections instead of binary sections will guide the reconstruction to get an approximated volume. However, only by adding 3-dimensional information in the form of the MRI volume, which acts as an undistorted reference, is an accurate reconstruction possible. A more detailed analysis of this issue can be found in [24].

---

[3] Neuroimaging Informatics Technology Initiative (NIfTI) : http://nifti.nimh.nih.gov

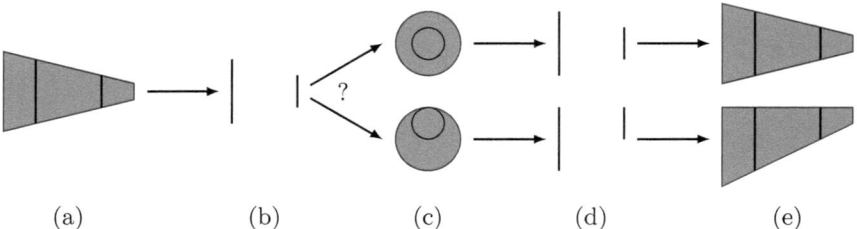

Figure 2.9 The 2-dimensional registration method may affect the spatial geometry of an object. Sketch (a) illustrates a binary 3-dimensional shape, which is drawn from a sagittal view. If the object is cut in frontal sections (b) as it happens in histology only the 2-dimensional information of the sections are available. It is uncertain what the correct alignment of the frontal sections should be ((c) frontal view, (d) sagittal view). Depending on the 2-dimensional registration the resulting 3-dimensional volume could differ (e).

2.4 Co-Registration of Fluorescent Histology Images and MR Images

Once the 3-dimensional histology volume is reconstructed it can be co-registered with the MRI volume. From here on, a volume is defined as an image (see definition in section 2.2.1) with dimension $d = 3$. During the registration process the MRI volume represents the reference R and the histology volume the template T. This implies that the MRI volume will not be transformed and therefore the structure and shape of the volume will be preserved. Note that a slice-to-slice correspondence is scarcely to be expected since the thickness of slices differ in MRI and histology. The histology slices have a thickness of 50 μm. However, due to the fact that only every tenth slice is available for processing a thickness of 500 μm is assumed. Note that the MRI slices have a thickness of 600 μm. Likewise, in general, it is not to be presumed that the histology sections are cut in the same angle as the MRI slices are acquired.

The co-registration follows the pipeline that is illustrated in figure 2.10. This multi-registration strategy consists of three consecutive alignment steps where each of the steps will converge to a more accurate alignment.

An initial alignment is performed by once again using the centre of mass P_{COM} as defined in formula 2.2. Phase two of the multi-registration approach makes use of the rigid transformation defined in formula 2.4. The result of this registration step is used as an initial transformation for further alignments as described in section 2.4.1.

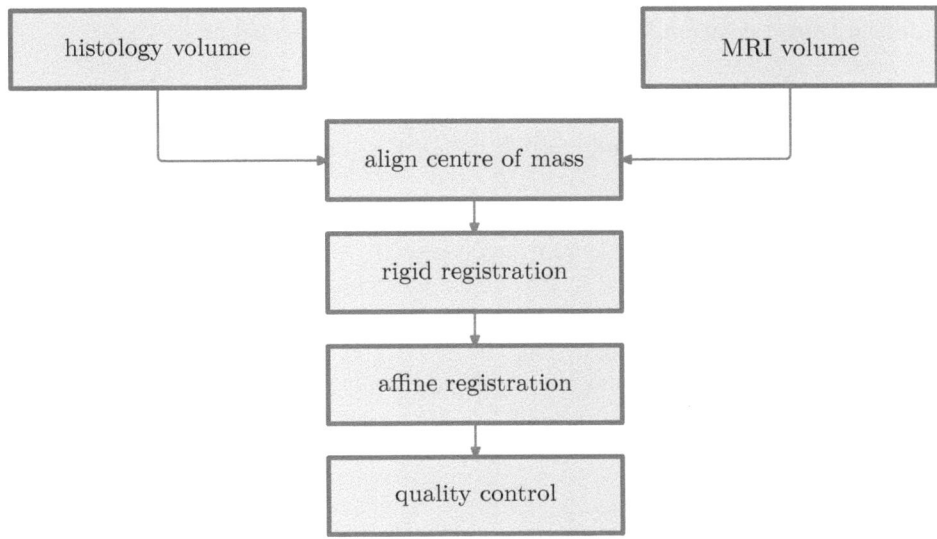

Figure 2.10 Pipeline for the 3-dimensional co-registration of the MRI volume and the histology volume.

Since the SSD measure is not feasible for the multimodal registration problem a different distance measure that is defined in section 2.4.2 is applied. Once more, the optimisation method introduced by Klein et al. [34] is adopted. Note that, due to the stochastic approach of the optimisation (see section 2.3.4) only a subset of spatial points that are selected on a grid are used for the co-registration. This method reduces the computational cost for the images rapidly.

A multi-resolution approach with a Gaussian pyramid ($\sigma = 4.0, 2.0, 1.0$ voxel) as described in section 2.3.5 is used for the rigid and affine registration. Note that no down-sampling is performed in this multi-resolution strategy since the in-vivo MR scans of the animals already have a poor resolution.

2.4.1 Affine Transformation

Investigations in the literature have shown that an affine transformation is suitable for the proposed registration problem [15, 21 and 24]. An affine transformation allows an optimisation in respect to translation, rotation, shearing, and scaling. This allows the registration not only to align the histology volume to the MRI but to correct distortions that are caused during the cutting process and shrinking of the tissue that may occur over time. Hence, the third phase of the proposed pipeline is based on an affine registration, which uses the result of the rigid registration as an initial transformation. An affine transformation is defined as

$$\varphi(x) = Ax + b \tag{2.12}$$

with $A \in \mathbb{R}^{d \times d}$, $det\, A > 0$ and $b = \mathbb{R}^d$. Since $d = 3$ the registration has 12 degrees of freedom.

2.4.2 Normalised Mutual Information

Since the SSD distance measure is based on the assumption that the same anatomical area in two different images has the same grey values it is not feasible for a multimodal registration. A more suitable approach would assume that a region of similar tissue in one image with a specific grey value distribution corresponds to a region in another image that has a similar distribution even though the grey values may differ.

Mutual information (MI) only assumes a probabilistic relationship between intensities and has shown to be an accurate distance measure for the registration of medical images [36]. First introduced by Woods et al. [37 and 38] for multimodal registration problems MI is now widely used in the literature for MRI and light microscopy registration [15] or determination of histology and MRI correspondence [19 and 21].

MI is a entropy-based measure that is originated in information theory. The precise definition of the distance measure $\mathcal{D}^{MI} : \mathbb{R}^{2d} \to \mathbb{R}$ can be written as

$$\mathcal{D}^{MI}(R, T) = H(\rho_R) + H(\rho_T) - H(\rho_{R,T}) \tag{2.13}$$

where $H(x)$ denotes the entropy and ρ_R, ρ_T, and $\rho_{R,T}$ the grey value densities of R, T and the joined grey value distribution, respectively. Since MI measures the entropy of the joint density it is maximal if the images are maximally related. In 1999 Studholme [39] showed that with increasing misalignment the MI may actually increase. This could be due to the fact that the marginal entropies may increase faster than the joint entropy when the relative areas of object and background even out. In order to solve this issue a normalised measure of mutual information [39] was proposed, which is less sensitive to changes in overlap:

$$\mathcal{D}^{NMI}(R, T) = \frac{H(\rho_R) + H(\rho_T)}{H(\rho_{R,T})}. \tag{2.14}$$

Normalised mutual information (NMI) has proven to be a qualified distance measure for the proposed co-registration of MRI and fluorescent histology image data.

2.4.3 Interpolation

After the 3-dimensional reconstruction the histology volume has a dimension of around 1388 px × 1040 px × 22 px, which differs from the size of the MRI volume. During the co-registration and therefore the comparison of histology and MRI it may happen that the distance measure needs to be evaluated at non-voxel positions. For that reason the volume needs to be interpolated based on the dimension of the corresponding MRI volume. Note that the MRI is already upsampled with a factor of 10 (see section 2.2.2) such that the grid matrix that can be used to evaluate the distance measure has a size of approximately 620 × 440 × 23. In order to evaluate the histology volume on the same grid matrix a linear interpolation is applied. Here, the intensity of a non-voxel position is the weighted average of the surrounding voxels where weight is based on the distance to each voxel. This linear interpolation approach gives satisfying results in terms of computation time and quality during the registration process.

If the registration is finished the final transformation is applied to the histology volume. Since computation time is not as important as during the registration and quality has a much higher weight a 3rd-order b-spline interpolation is used in order to acquire the resulting histology volume. This type of interpolation is constructing new data points by using piecewise cubic polynomial between known data points.

2.5 Validation Based on Landmarks

Experts of the Institute of Psychiatry, King's College London defined anatomical landmarks based on structures like corpus callosum, ventricles, or anterior commissure. For each animal a set of 20 to 25 points were selected for the MRI volume and the histology volume. Landmarks were first defined in one modality before the corresponding points were defined in the non-registered associated image data. In figure 2.11 a subset of landmarks for the MRI volume and the corresponding non-registered histology data is presented. In row one sections of MRI and histology (position relative to bregma[4] ca. 2.76 mm) are shown with landmarks describing the anterior commissure (anterior part). Row two illustrates sections (bregma ca. 1.20 mm) with landmarks on the edge of the corpus callosum and the ventricles. Sections (bregma ca. -0.36 mm) with landmarks at the corpus callosum and the anterior commissure are shown in row three. Row four and five shows again landmarks near the corpus callosum.

The challenge to find corresponding points is massively affected by the relatively low quality of the MR image data. Therefore anatomical features are chosen that are well recognisable in both imaging modalities.

2.6 Registration Parameters

The proposed imaging pipeline was developed under the use of the image registration toolkit elastix [29], which allows the user to easily configure own registration methods. The toolkit is based on the insight segmentation and registration toolkit (ITK) and is distributed under the BSD license approved by the Open Source Initiative (OSI)[5].

An overview of the experimentally determined parameters for the 3-dimensional reconstruction of the histology volume and its co-registration with the MRI volume is given in the following three tables (parameters for the reconstruction in table 2.1, the initial and final parameters for the co-registration in table 2.2 and table 2.3, respectively). The parameters are carefully chosen in a sensible range and tested on image data of three animals. As it is shown in chapter 3 these parameters are particularly suited for an accurate 3-dimensional reconstruction of a histology volume and a precise co-registration with the corresponding MRI volume.

---

[4] Bregma is a reference point on the skull of the rat brain that is most commonly used as a reference point for stereotaxic surgery.
[5] http://www.opensource.org/licenses/bsd-license.php

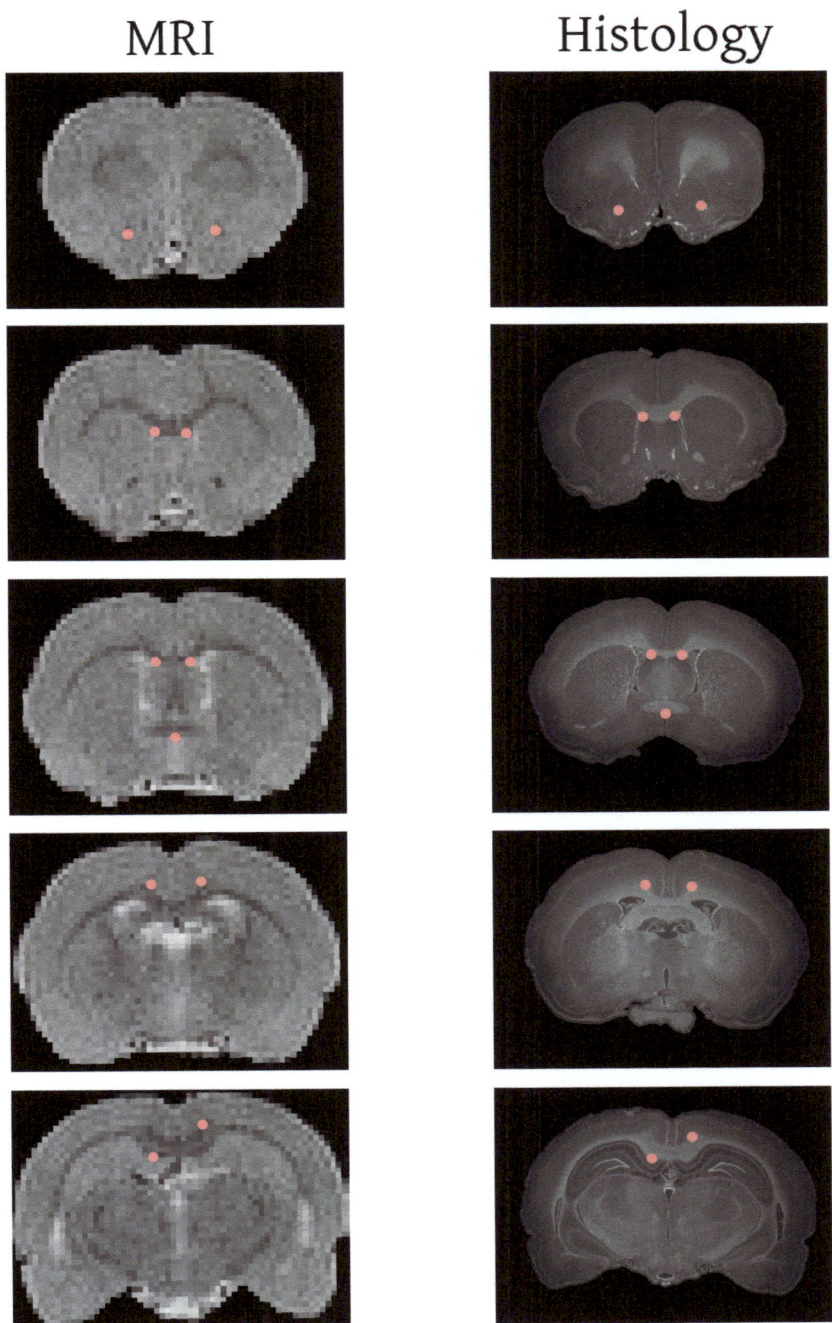

Figure 2.11 Corresponding anatomical landmarks in MRI (slice 5, 6, 9, 11, and 16) and Histology (slice 2, 4, 7, 9, and 15) before registration.

registration parameter	value
dimension	2
transformation	rigid
degrees of freedom	3
distance measurement	SSD
number of histogram bins	256
multi-resolution	true
number of resolutions	2
B-spline interpolation order	3
optimiser	ASGD
max. number of iterations	300
max. step length	5.0
number of spatial samples	10
image sampler	grid

Table 2.1 Registration parameters for the 3-dimensional reconstruction of the histology volume as described in section 2.3.

registration parameter	value
dimension	3
transformation	rigid
degrees of freedom	6
distance measurement	NMI
number of histogram bins	64
multi-resolution	false
B-spline interpolation order	3
optimiser	ASGD
max. number of iterations	300
max. step length	1.0
number of spatial samples	10000
image sampler	grid

Table 2.2 Registration parameters for the initial co-registration of the histology and MRI volume as described in section 2.4.

registration parameter	value
dimension	3
transformation	affine
degrees of freedom	12
distance measurement	NMI
number of histogram bins	64
multi-resolution	true
number of resolutions	2
B-spline interpolation order	3
optimiser	ASGD
max. number of iterations	200
max. step length	0.5
number of spatial samples	10000
image sampler	grid

Table 2.3 Registration parameters for the final co-registration of the histology and MRI volume as described in section 2.4.

3
Results

The following chapter will cover the results of the proposed imaging pipeline. In section 3.1 the 3-dimensional reconstructed histology volume is illustrated and discussed. The results of the co-registration of the histology and MRI volume are shown in section 3.2. A detailed analysis of the quality in terms of the alignment of corresponding anatomical features is presented in section 3.2.1. Since the imaging pipeline is developed with respect to a particular image set from a group of three animals (training set), the proposed method is applied to additional image data (validation set) in order to validate consistency over multiple data sets (section 3.2.2). In section 3.2.3 the applicability of the co-registration for microstructural analysis is discussed. Finally, the imaging pipeline is tested on abnormal image data and is applied to fluorescent histology and MR images of rats that suffered a stroke (stroke set)–the results are presented in section 3.2.4.

3.1 Reconstruction of Histology Volume

All experiments were performed on a Mac Pro with 32 GB memory and 12 cores at 2536 MHz on Mac OS X 10.6.8(x64). The average computation time of the 2-dimensional registration of two images amounts to 54.3 seconds. Since it is necessary to perform about 22 registrations for the reconstruction of a whole volume, the time for the 3-dimensional reconstruction totals up to about 20 minutes. Note that the time to compute the overall transformation for each section takes less than a second and is therefore not taken into account. A way how the reconstruction of the histology volume can be speeded up is discussed in section 4.2.1.

In figure 3.1 the horizontal and sagittal plane of the unregistered and registered histology image stack is presented. The image data is based on DAPI stained tissue.

Note that as a result of an acquisition of histology images with respect to the reconstruction, the tissue sections are approximately centred (by eye) in the middle of the images (compare with figure 2.3). Therefore it is easy to guess the shape of the brain by looking at the unregistered image stack. The sagittal view (figure 3.1(b)) indicates a misalignment of the images due to certain slices. No anatomical structures are discernible in this view plane. In the horizontal view (figure 3.1 (a)) the hippocampus (two dark, almost rhomboid-shaped structures in the upper half of figure 3.1(c) labeled h) can be estimated but the shape stays unrecognisable.

After applying the proposed imaging pipeline for reconstruction of the fluorescent histology volume the hippocampus and its shape is clearly identifiable (figure 3.1(c)). Furthermore, detailed structures like the corpus callosum (bright border around the hippocampus, labeled cc in figure 3.1 (c)) or the granular layer of the dentate gyrus (bright area inside the left part of the hippocampus, labeled dg in figure 3.1(c)) are recognisable. Moreover, these anatomical features are also visible in the sagittal plane of the registered image stack.

Considering the surface of the image stack in horizontal and sagittal view after reconstruction, one can obtain a smooth shape of the brain. Especially no more misaligned slices that stick out of the volume are detectable. A more profound impression of the shape can be gained by studying the 2-dimensional projection of the 3-dimensional reconstructed rat brain in figure 3.2. While the unregistered image stack in figure 3.2(a)-(c) shows a blurred and irregular surface one can obtain the typical form of the 3-dimensional body of a rat brain in the reconstructed volume (figure 3.2(d)-(e)). Macroscopic visible details like the longitudinal cerebral fissure or the cerebral hemispheres are clearly recognisable. Even though, the shape of the volume cannot be considered as spatial correct before a registration with an undistorted reference volume is performed (see co-registration with MRI in section 2.4 and section 3.2) gives the reconstructed histology volume already a good approximation for the spatial orientation of anatomical features. The same results as here elucidated were found quantitatively over all used image sets, too. Note that a reasonable 3-dimensional reconstruction is required for a robust co-registration of the histology and MRI volume as it is presented in the following section.

3.2 Co-Registration of Fluorescent Histology Images and MR Images

After reconstruction of the histology volume, the co-registration with the MRI volume is performed on the same machine as described before (Mac Pro, 32 GB memory, 12 cores at 2536 MHz, Mac OS X 10.6.8(x64)). Following an initial alignment of

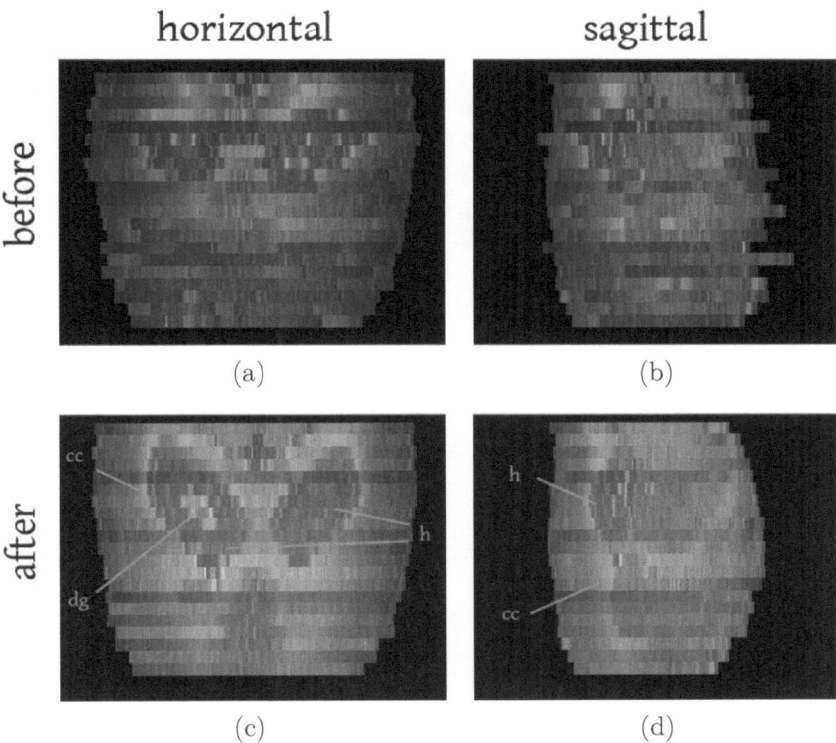

Figure 3.1 Horizontal and sagittal view of the fluorescent histology image stack before and after registration. (a) horizontal plane of the non-registered volume. (b) sagittal plane of the non-registered volume. (c) horizontal plane of the volume after reconstruction. (d) sagittal plane of the volume after reconstruction. Anatomical features like the hippocampus (h), corpus callosum (cc), or dentate gyrus (dg) are clearly recognisable after 3-dimensional reconstruction of the histology images.

histology volume and MRI volume, a co-registration under the use of a rigid transformation was applied. The registration was performed using the up-sampled MRI volume with a resolution that averages 620 px × 440 px × 23 px (equals 6274400 voxels). This performance took around 4.56 minutes on the three different animals that are used in order to develop the proposed imaging pipeline. Adopting the result of the rigid registration as an initial transformation, the affine registration was applied. This registration step, which uses a multi-resolution approach with three different resolutions, took on average 8.34 minutes. Accordingly, the overall time for the co-registration of histology and MRI takes around 13 minutes.

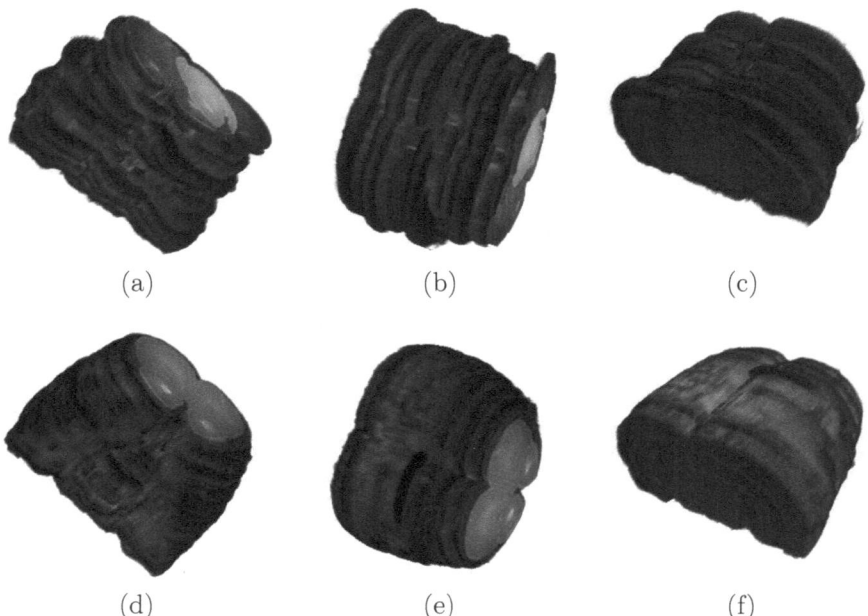

Figure 3.2 Overview of the 3-dimensional reconstruction of non-registered and registered fluorescent image stack. Image (a), (b), and (c) shows the view from below, above and from the back of the non-registered volume. Image (d), (e), and (f) shows the volume after the 2-dimensional registration process, respectively.

In figure 3.3 the MRI volume and the corresponding histology volume is presented after the proposed imaging pipeline is applied. The volumes are plotted in the frontal, horizontal, and sagittal plane from top to bottom. The red cross indicates the position of associated planes. The right column shows the histology volume superimposed on the MRI with an opacity of 50%. It is clearly visible that the surface of the MRI and histology volume match. The results of the proposed imaging pipeline shows that the histology volume is spatially aligned at the anatomical correct position with reference to the MRI volume. Note that the used affine registration was able to correct shrinkage and distortions of the histology sections that may occur during the sectioning, immunohistochemistry, and mounting process. Since MRI preserves the physical structure of the object, except from some artefacts caused by inhomogeneity of the main magnet [40], the histology volume can now be considered as correctly anatomically shaped.

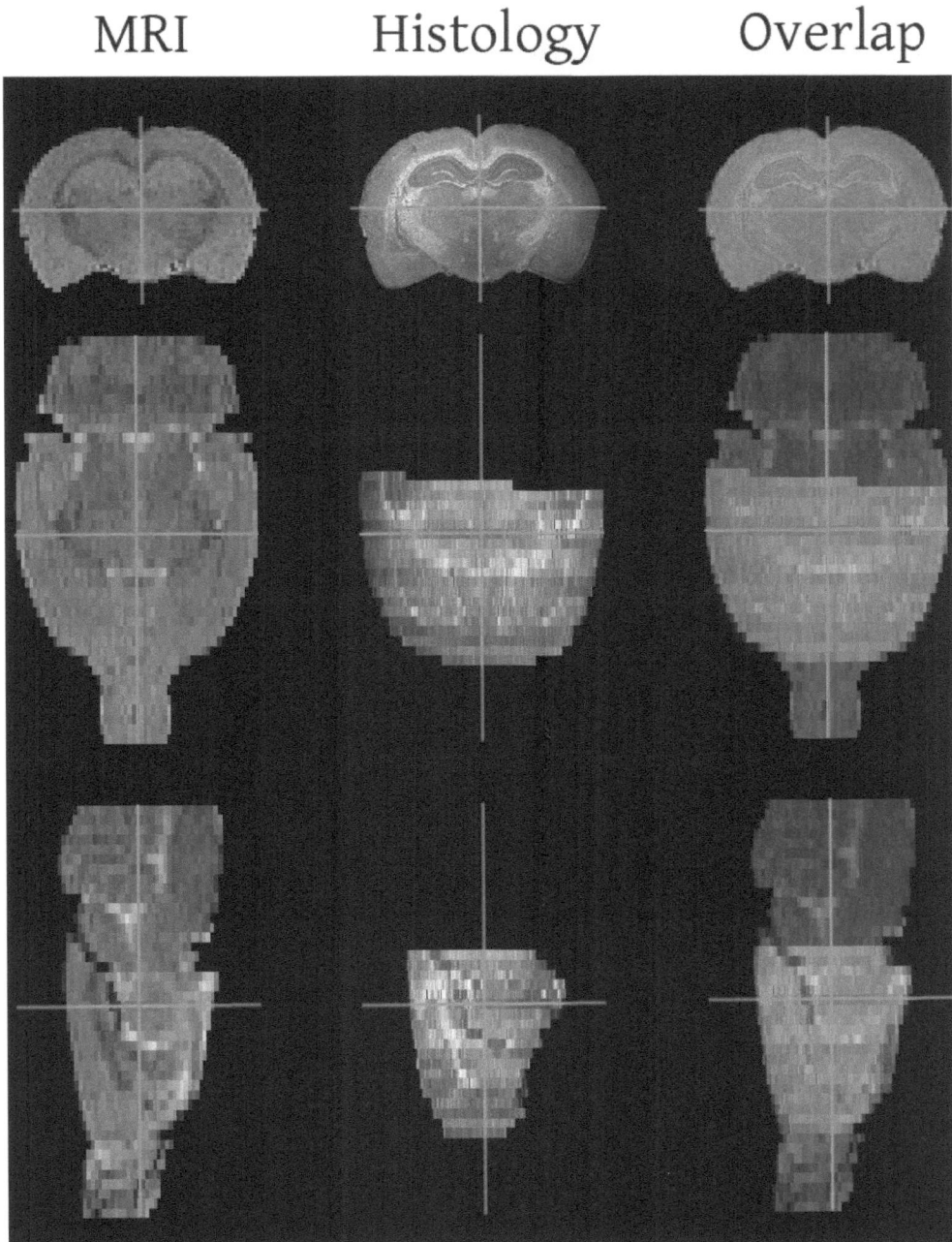

Figure 3.3 Frontal, horizontal, and sagittal view of the MR volume and the histology volume. Column one shows the MR volume, column two shows the histology volume and column three shows the histology volume superimposed on the MR volume with an opacity of 50%.

Note that a histology slice after co-registration does not necessarily correspond to a slice in the histology image stack before co-registration. Once the final transformation is applied the histology volume is translated, rotated, scaled, and sheared in three dimensions. However, in order to study frontal slices of the volume as they are often investigated in neuroscience, a frontal cut through the histology volume is performed based on the orientation of the MRI slices to generate spatially equivalent histology slices. The cuts are computed using a 3rd-order B-spline interpolation as described in section 2.4.3.

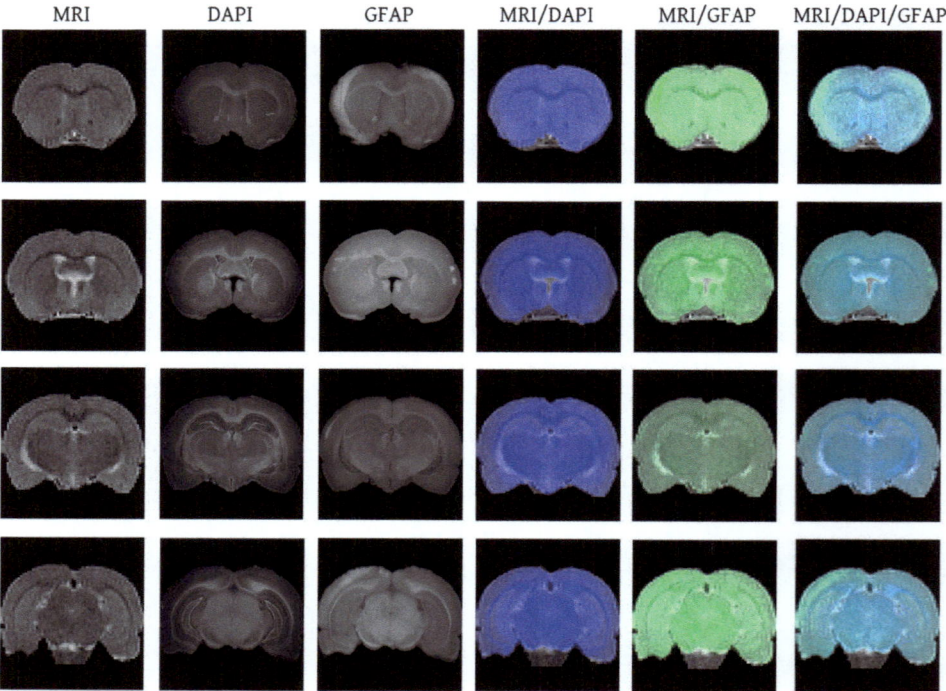

Figure 3.4 Overlay of different fluorescent histology stains on MRI. Column one shows frontal slices of the MRI. Column two and three shows corresponding histology slice with a DAPI and a GFAP staining. In column four and five the overlay of the DAPI and GFAP staining on the MRI can be observed, respectively. Column six illustrates the combination of the DAPI and GFAP staining superimposed on the MRI. Row 1-4 shows frontal slices at different positions along the rat brain (row 1: interaural 9.6 mm, bregma 0.6 mm; row 2: interaural 8.0 mm, bregma -1.0 mm; row 3: interaural 5.3 mm, bregma -3.7 mm; row 4: interaural 3.0 mm, bregma -6.0 mm)

Figure 3.4 shows high-resolution histology sections superimposed on the corresponding MRI slices. Since it is possible to acquire histology images of different stains in the same space, the same transformation can be used to align the specific image data with the MRI volume. Therefore, the imaging pipeline only needs to be applied once and no additional time is required. The resulting histology image sets can be used to study the correlation of multiple features of interest with the corresponding MRI volume. This is among other things beneficial in the research of degenerative diseases like Alzheimer's or Parkinson's where an investigation of certain stains is necessary. In figure 3.4 histology sections with a DAPI-staining and a GFAP-staining along with the MRI volume are illustrated. Each row shows sections of a different position along the rat brain. The structures obtained are with reference to bregma at 0.6 mm, -1.0 mm, -3.7 mm, and -6.0 mm. The shapes of the histology sections are aligned on the MRI such that the surface of the two modalities match. Obtaining the anatomy seen in the sections, a correspondence of hippocampus, ventricle, and corpus callosum can be considered as consistent because their position is defined with respect to areas visible in both modalities, which are well-registered under an affine transformation. The superimposition of the histology images over the MRI slices shows that it is now possible to localise anatomical structures that were almost undetectable in the MRI volume before the imaging pipeline was applied.

3.2.1 Evaluation Based on Anatomical Landmarks

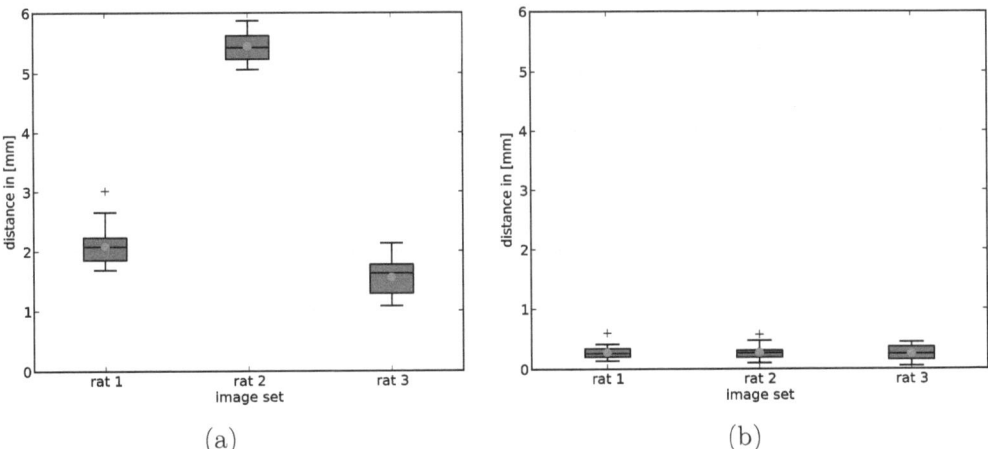

Figure 3.5 The distances between anatomical landmarks in MRI and histology for the training set before (a) and after (b) registration. The black cross indicates outliers and the red dot indicates the mean of the distances for each image set.

image set	rigid transformation	affine transformation
rat 1	0.581	0.277
rat 2	0.435	0.266
rat 3	0.562	0.255

Table 3.1 The mean distance of landmarks after rigid and affine transformation in [mm]. A consistent improvement from rigid to affine registration is observable.

Once the anatomical landmarks are defined (see section 2.5) and the proposed imaging pipeline is applied, the distance between the landmarks can be determined. Figure 3.5 illustrates a box- and-whisker plot of the distances between landmarks that are previously defined for the three animals that are used in order to develop the imaging pipeline. The smallest observation, lower quartile, median, upper quartile, and largest observation is presented. The red dot is related with the mean value. Outliers are indicated by crosses. In figure 3.5(a) the distances of landmarks before co-registration are shown while the distances after co-registration are presented in figure 3.5(b). A decrease of error distances between corresponding landmarks after co-registration is clearly noticeable. While the distances before co-registration are arbitrary, afterwards corresponding points are correct aligned with an mean error of 0.266 mm. This is consistent with the MRI in-plane voxel dimension of 0.234 mm.

In table 3.1 the progression of error distances is presented. While after co-registration with a rigid transformation a error of around 0.526 mm is detectable, the following affine registration leads to an almost halved error of 0.266 mm (mean values). This indicates a sub-voxel accuracy considering the space diagonal of a voxel in the MRI volume of 0.685 mm.

Figure 3.6 illustrates the error distances relative to the position along the rat brain. In order to determine the position of the landmarks bregma is used as a point of reference. The variation of distances between corresponding landmarks displays a nearly uniform distribution along the brain. It is noteworthy that the cause for some slightly deviant error distances between landmarks in the front of the brain near the olfactory bulb and the posterior part of the brain are probably due to errors made by the user and/or the fact that anatomical structures used for landmarks are hard to perceive. For instance, the forceps minor of the corpus callosum is visible in MRI and histology, but serves inconclusive information for landmarks since the boundaries are vague (see first row in figure 2.11).

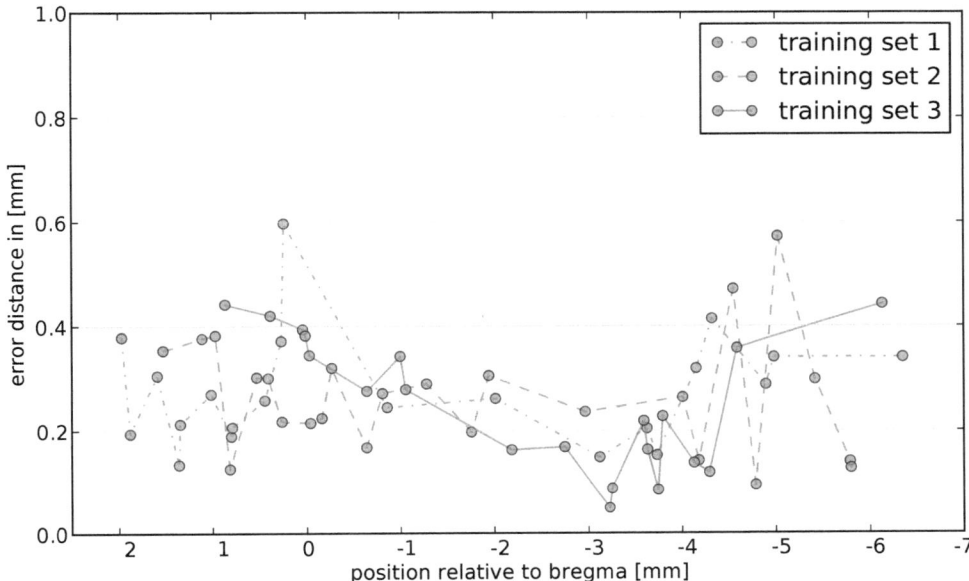

Figure 3.6 Distances between anatomical landmarks in MRI and histology relative to bregma. Error distances are almost uniform along the brain.

3.2.2 Validation with Additional Animals

Up to this point, it is shown that the proposed co-registration works for the three animals that are used in order to develop the imaging pipeline. An alignment measurement based on manually selected anatomical landmarks indicates an error of 0.266 mm. In order to prove that the co-registration gives similar results for previously unseen animals, additional experiments were performed. The images for three more animals were acquired using the same techniques as described in section 2.1. Again, at least 20 corresponding landmarks were defined for each data set. Figure 3.7 illustrates the distances of landmarks after co-registration compared to the three animals used for the development of the imaging pipeline. It is without any doubt recognisable that the proposed 3-dimensional reconstruction and following co-registration delivers comparable results for animals that were not available during the development. While the first three animals show an error of 0.266 mm, a mean error of 0.249 mm can be detected for animals that were previously unseen. This clearly indicates that the distances between landmarks is similar across different animals and shows that the proposed imaging pipeline is performs consistently.

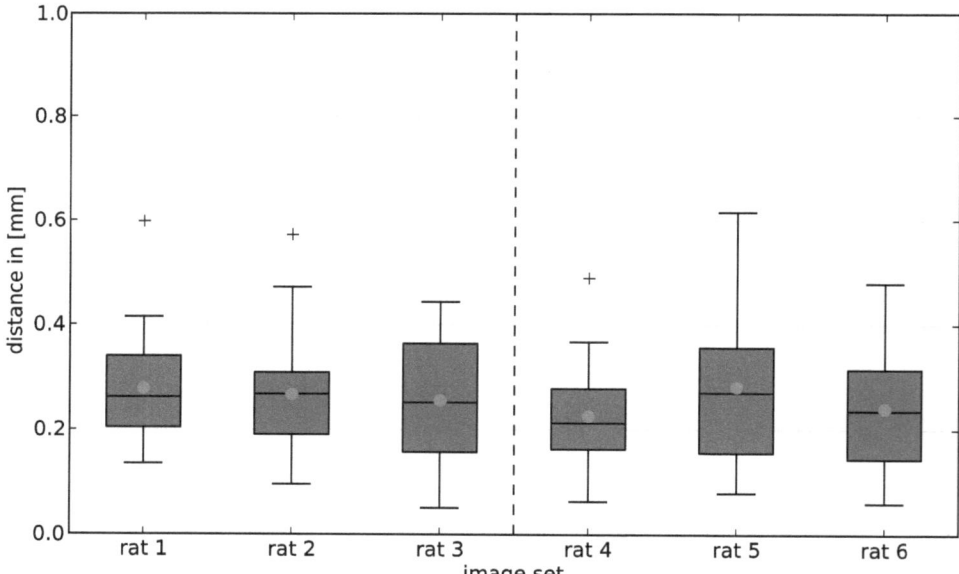

Figure 3.7 The errors distance between anatomical landmarks in the MRI and the histology for the training set (rat 1, 2, and 3) and the validation set (rat 4, 5, and 6). The black cross indicates outliers and the red dot indicates the mean of the distances for each image set.

The distances of corresponding landmarks with respect to its position along the brain of the validation group indicate comparable results with the training group (figure 3.8). Again a slight increase of error distances in the front of the brain is observable (see page 38 for a more detailed analysis of this issue).

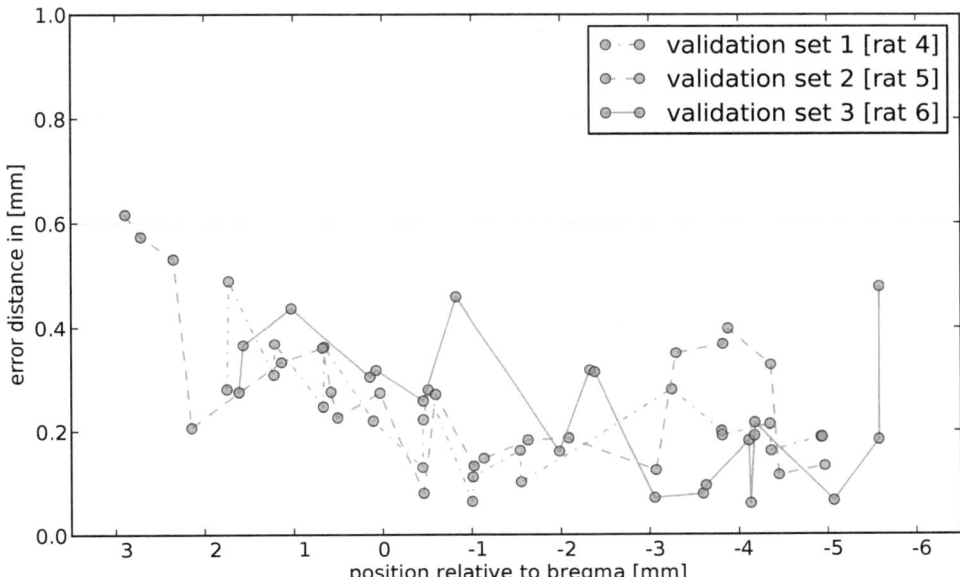

Figure 3.8 Distances between anatomical landmarks in MRI and histology relative to bregma of the validation image sets. See figure 3.6 for comparison.

In table 3.2 the mean distances between corresponding landmarks of the training group and the validation group is presented. No significant difference between the two groups is recognisable. The validation group displays similar results after affine registration as the test group. It is noteworthy that even an insufficient alignment after initial rigid registration (e.g. rat 6 with an error of 0.732 mm) leads to an accurate matching of anatomical features after affine registration (0.240 mm). Taking all six animals into account, the mean error between corresponding landmarks amounts to 0.258 mm. This value indicates that even small structures visible in the tissue are matched up between MRI and histology and that a microstructural analysis of anatomical features is possible.

image set	rigid transformation	affine transformation
rat 1 (training)	0.581	0.277
rat 2 (training)	0.435	0.266
rat 3 (training)	0.562	0.255
rat 4 (validation)	0.412	0.226
rat 5 (validation)	0.524	0.281
rat 6 (validation)	0.732	0.240

Table 3.2 Mean distance of landmarks after rigid and affine transformation in [mm].

3.2.3 Microstructural Analysis of Anatomical Features

The evaluation of the co-registration under the use of anatomical landmarks selected by experts shows that the proposed imaging pipeline leads to an alignment that has an mean accuracy of 0.258 mm, which corresponds roughly to the in-plane resolution of 0.234 mm per pixel edge length in the MRI.

Sprague Dawley rats that are used in this study have a dorsoventral distance between the interaural line and bregma of 10.1 ± 0.1 mm [41]. The thickness of structures of interest vary between corpus callosum 0.42 mm (position relative to bregma 0.0 mm, lateral position 0.0 mm), hippocampus 1.8 mm (bregma -3.6 mm, lateral 3.0 mm), or the cerebral cortex 2.0 mm (bregma -3.2 mm, lateral 2.0 mm) [41]. This indicates that the precision of the proposed method enables an accurate study of microstructural features seen in histology and superimposed on the MRI.

Figure 3.9 shows a region of interest in MRI and histology that contains parts of hippocampus and corpus callosum. The position of the slice is approximately -3.36 mm with bregma as a reference point. The presented histology section that is stained with DAPI gives detailed information about the cell population in specific areas. This makes it possible to differentiate small anatomical structures like the corpus callosum, oriens layer, pyramidal cell layer, radiatum layer, or the lacunosum moleculare layer of the hippocampus. The overlay of the co-registered histology allows a detailed analysis of these areas in the MRI volume. Note that small structures are initially not visible in the volume on account of the relatively low resolution of the MRI.

Furthermore, it is possible to study brain tissue with additional stains that are acquired in connection with the DAPI stained sections (i.e. they are acquired in the same space as the DAPI stained sections with the result that the same transformations can be used for the co-registration). For instance, the GFAP stained tissue can be studied, which plays an important role in the research of Alzheimer's [42 and 43] or Parkinson's [44 and 45] disease, as well as in the research of stem cell transplantation and stroke [46].

In figure 3.9 the DAPI and GFAP stained histology sections are superimposed on the MRI using a pseudo colouring and an opacity of 50%. The colours are adjusted to the original frequency that is detected by the fluorescence microscope. The superimposition enables, for example, the creation of a microstructural atlas that can be applied to the MRI volume after co-registration. This would gain a more comprehensive understanding of anatomical and pathological structures [22, 47 and 48].

3.2.4 Validation with Animals Models of Stroke

The image data for three animals that suffered a stroke were acquired and the volume of the stroke lesions were manually measured (rat 7 : 40.947 μm^3; rat 8 : 34.4085 μm^3; rat 9 : 122.6765 μm^3). The same imaging pipeline that was applied to the healthy animals was adapted. It is noteworthy that no additional masking was performed in order to exclude the pathological structures. In figure 3.10 the results based on evaluation with anatomical landmarks are presented. At least 20 and up to 25 landmarks were defined for each set of images. For the three animals that suffered a stroke a mean error distance of 0.323 mm is observable. Comparing this with the results regarding the control group animals, which showed an error distance between corresponding landmarks of 0.258 mm, it is worth taking into consideration that a stronger distinction between MRI and histology is observable in the images. This may be due to significant deformations in areas affected by the stroke and the fact that the rigid and affine registration use a global transformation model, which do not represent localised deformations.

Figure 3.11 indicates that no difference in the error distances of landmarks with respect to the position along the brain is observable. Mentionable are the two outliers around position -1.0 mm with respect to bregma of rat 9. The large distance between corresponding landmarks in this area is caused by misregistration in the 3-dimensional reconstruction of the histology volume due to highly distorted tissue on account of the strong impact of the stroke in this part of the brain.

In figure 3.12 the co-registration result of rat 9 is illustrated. The presented MRI and histology sections are located at around -0.24 mm with respect to bregma. The decrease of blood flow in the right hemisphere leads to a decline of glucose and oxygen availability to neurons, which quickly results in neuronal death. The impact

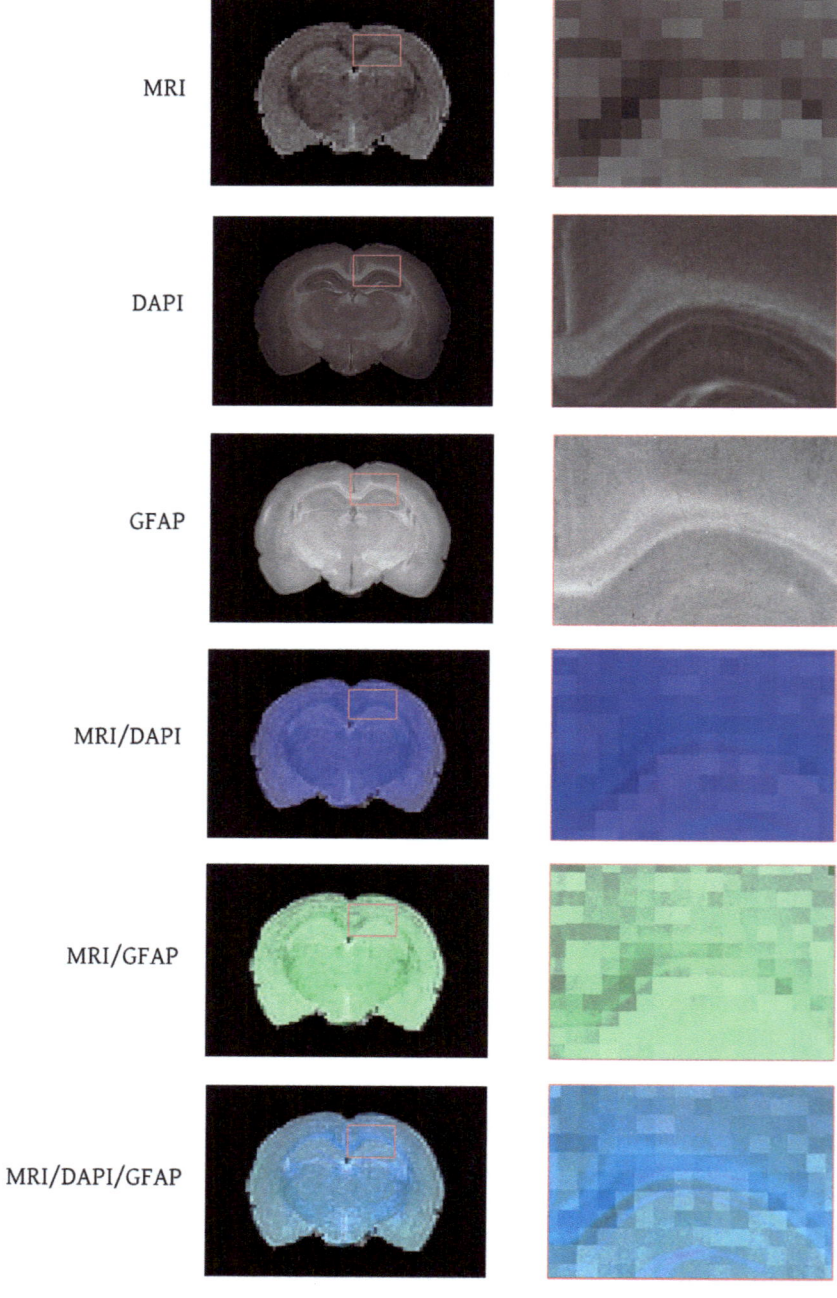

Figure 3.9 Axial plane of a registered MRI volume and histology volume. The region of interest shows details of the corpus callosum and the hippocampus. The registration enables a mapping of anatomical features seen in the fluorescent histology images to the MRI. Position of the sections relative to bregma is approximately -3.36 mm.

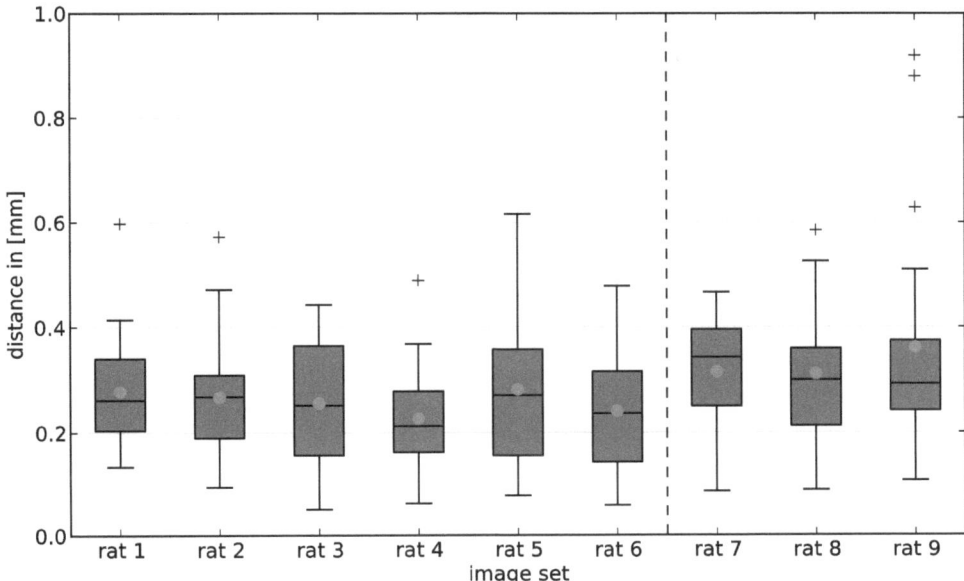

Figure 3.10 The error distances between anatomical landmarks in MRI and histology for control animals (rat 1 to 6) and animals that have suffered a stroke (rat 7 to 9). The black cross indicates outliers and the red dot indicates the mean of the distances for each image set.

of the stroke is clearly visible in the MRI by the hyperintense region in the right hemisphere (left side in the image). Shape and dimension of the pathological region is examinable. However, a detailed analysis of the necrotic tissue is first enabled by the superimposition of histology over the MRI. The correspondence between MRI and histology gives concrete information of deformations and damage of the tissue. The overlay of GFAP stained tissue allows an accurate investigation of glia scarring around the lesion [46] in the MRI volume.

Furthermore, this research contributes to the analysis of significant neuronal diseases and may effects the treatment of patients.

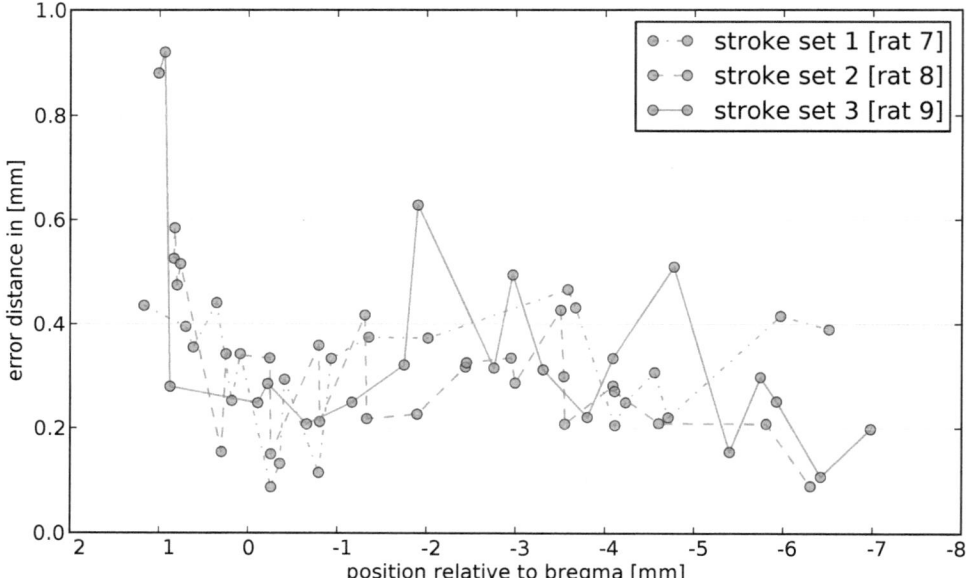

Figure 3.11 Distances between anatomical landmarks in MRI and histology relative to bregma after co-registration from animals that have suffered a stroke.

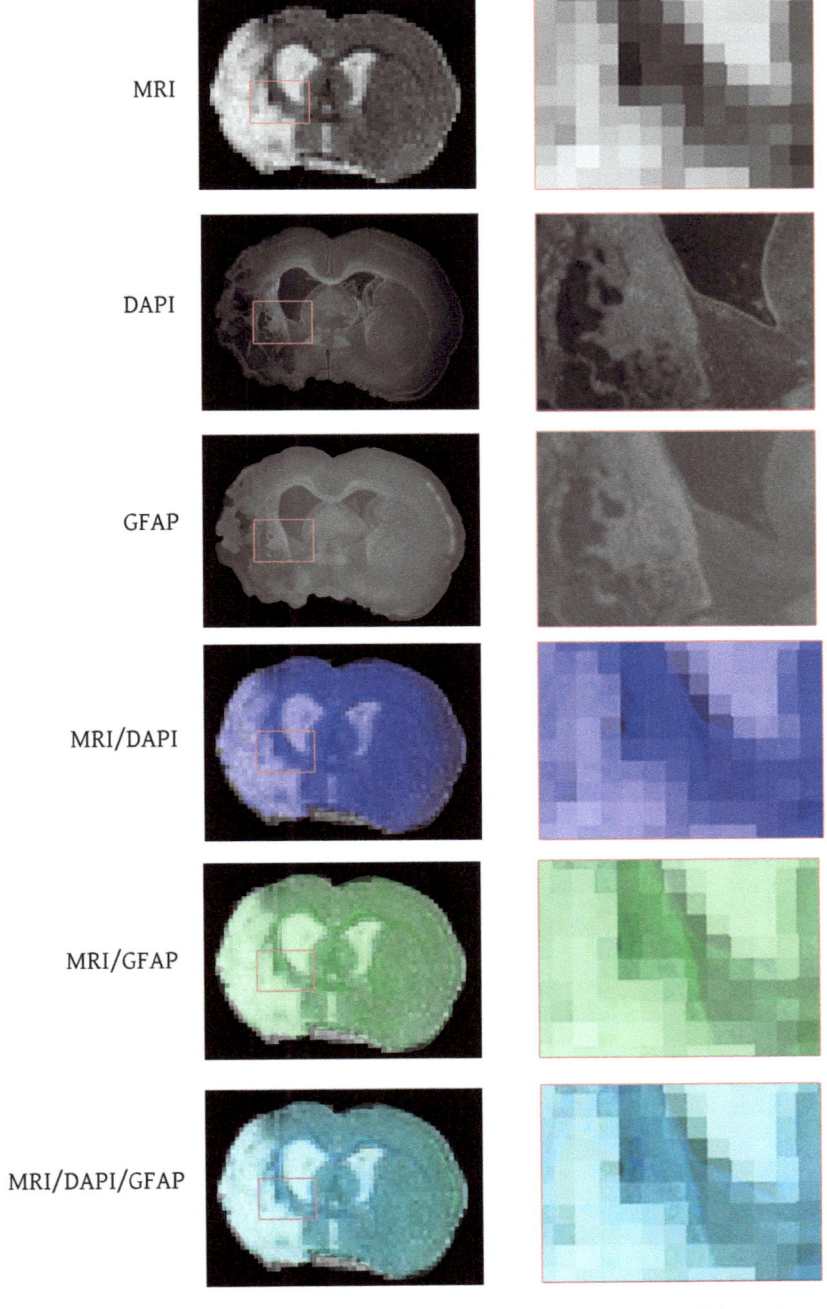

Figure 3.12 Axial plane of a registered MRI volume and histology volume. The region of interest shows details of a stroke in the right hemisphere. The registration enables a mapping of anatomical features seen in the fluorescent histology images to the MRI.

4
Discussion

In the previous chapter the evaluation of the proposed imaging pipeline is described. A training image data set of three rat brains were used in order to develop and test the proposed imaging pipeline iteratively until an accuracy of 0.266 mm is reached and a microstructural analysis is enabled. In order to prove constant performance, the imaging pipeline was applied to an additional validation image set, which consisted of three animals. The evaluation of the validation set resulted in an accuracy of 0.249 mm and therefore showed consistently accurate alignment of the histology to the MRI volume. After proving that the proposed method works on normal data it is applied to abnormal data. A set of three animals that suffered a stroke was used to evaluate the performance on image data that features pathological and destructed structures in the tissue. Again, the proposed imaging pipeline led to an exact alignment of 0.323 mm and showed that even if abnormal local deformations occur, the affine registration is capable of aligning the histology image and the MRI correctly. Furthermore, the obtained accuracy is precise enough to allow experts a detailed comparison of histology and MR image data of normal and abnormal tissue.

Nevertheless, some factors that affect the registration process negatively are still present. Problems that may occur during the performance of the proposed imaging pipeline with normal and abnormal image data are discussed in section 4.1. This discussion is followed by an analysis of methods that potentially improve the here presented method. Section 4.3 will focus on methods and applications that could serve a potential extension of the proposed imaging pipeline.

4.1 Source of Errors

The following two sections will cover sources of error that may occur during the acquisition of images (section 4.1.1) and the evaluation of the proposed imaging pipeline (section 4.1.2).

4.1.1 Histology Image Data

Several exemplarily images are presented in this thesis (e.g. figure 2.3, figure 2.11, figure 3.3, figure 3.4, figure 3.9, or figure 3.12). An accurate and precise performance of the sectioning, immunohistochemistry, and mounting is fundamental in order to acquire usable histology images. Nevertheless, even if the procedure is performed by experienced neuroscientists some almost unavoidable artefacts may occur in the images. Most commonly, the images show cuts and holes that emerge during the cutting process of the 50 μm thin histology sections. In the worst case the tissue would tear apart in two independent parts. In order to correct this, one would have to put the individual pieces together during the mounting process, which will presumably result in a distorted tissue section. An automatic alternative was proposed by Schubert et al. in 2009 [49]. Fortunately, this issue did not appear during experiments due to the precise work of the neuroscientists that were involved in this project.

After all, the tissue is under a lot of strain while mounting the sections on a slide and a careful handling is essential. A problem that occasionally occurs while the mounted tissue is covered are folds. Small tissue folds are characterised by an overlap of tissue. Here, the correct intensity value of a pixel in this area is manipulated by another value that is added up. It is not possible for a transformation, where only the position of a pixel is changed but not the intensity value, to correct this kind of deformation. Therefore it is important to correct the folds manually before images of fluorescent histology sections are taken.

Another problem that may affect the registration process is the bleaching of stains. Over time a photochemical destruction of fluorophores takes place which complicates the observation of fluorescent molecules. It is possible to decrease the effect of photobleaching by reducing the intensity and time-span of the light exposure. With this in mind, the acquisition of the fluorescent images were performed in the dark. For the rest of the time, the slides were stored in a box that is impermeable to light. Since the acquisition of bright field images is necessary for the masking process the slides had to be exposed to light. In order to reduce the strain due to light, the exposure time was limited to 200 ms with a light spectrum of 2650 K.

However, even if a careful handling of the histology slides is taken in mind, an inhomogeneity of the intensity distribution in the fluorescent histology sections is still observable over time. Additionally, the intensity of the fluorescence can be negatively influenced by a misalignment of the light source. An irregular illumination of the specimen can lead to an unwanted weighting of regions of interest where underexposed areas may have less influence during registration process. Different methods can be found in the literature to correct this inhomogeneity problem [50–54]. Wirtz proposed a simultaneous intensity correction and registration of histology images where the inhomogeneity of the intensity distribution is compared with noise [9].

During the development of the imaging pipeline, an anisotropic diffusion smoothing is tested and applied to the histology images in order to correct small differences in the intensity distribution. Anisotropic diffusion smoothing preserves edges and is therefore suitable to reduce the noise and inhomogeneity in the images. However, no visible difference of the reconstructed histology volume could be found. A detailed analysis and comparison of the volume resulting from the smoothed images and the volume that results from the not smoothed images remains to be done.

Furthermore does the co-registration presumably benefit from an intensity normalisation over all histology images since a more consistent intensity distribution of an anatomical feature over the whole image stack would lead to a better correlation with the MRI.

4.1.2 Error of the Landmark based Evaluation

The landmark based evaluation gives a detailed analysis of the quality of the proposed imaging pipeline. A prerequisite is, however, that the anatomical features are clearly and precisely definable. As mentioned before (section 2.5 and section 3.2.1), this is not constantly the case. Furthermore, the accuracy of a selected landmark depends on the landmark size relative to the pixel size. Therefore, the relatively low quality of the MRI makes it difficult to define the location of some anatomical features exactly. The process is additionally complicated by the fact that some anatomical features do not have a well-defined border (e.g. forceps minor of the corpus callosum). The selection of anatomical landmarks is aggravated by the fact that no initially slice-to-slice correspondence of MRI and histology is observable. The corresponding point to a landmark that is selected in a slice of one imaging modality could potentially lay within the space of two consecutive slices in the other modality.

Since the definition of the landmarks is up to the neuroscientists discretion, the localisation is only as exact as far as it is humanly possible to tell. In order to validate the accuracy of the selected landmarks, the neuroscientists would have to define the same anatomical landmarks multiple times and the variance would need to be determined. However, due to a limitation of time for this project, the precision of the anatomical landmarks is not evaluated but is feasible in the future.

4.2 Potential Improvements of the Imaging Pipeline

In the present thesis an imaging pipeline for the reconstruction of a fluorescent histology volume and its co-registration with MRI is presented that has almost the accuracy of a pixel edge length of the MRI. However, there are still some improvements in terms of execution time and quality of the registration conceivable. In the following sections some of these points will be discussed.

4.2.1 Parallelism of the Imaging Pipeline

In section 3.1 is annotated that the reconstruction of a whole histology volume takes around 20 minutes. For the reconstruction, the 2-dimensional registration of ca. 22 consecutive histology sections is necessary. Since each of the 2-dimensional registrations are independent from the other ones, these registration steps can be performed simultaneously. This parallelisation of the 2-dimensional registration would speed up the time of the 3-dimensional reconstruction of the histology volume rapidly.

A parallelisation of the 3-dimensional co-registration, on the other hand, is in this respect not possible because the co-registration is based on one single registration step including two 3-dimensional volumes.

4.2.2 Additional Slice-to-Slice Registration

Xiao et al. [21] proposed an approach for the co-registration of histology and MRI that involved a 2-dimensional slice-to-slice registration of histology and MRI slices. The method improved iteratively the correspondence between histology and MRI by performing a 2-dimensional registration of estimated corresponding histology and MRI slices, generating a pseudo histology volume, performing a volume-to-volume registration and starting again until an optimal alignment is reached [21].

For the proposed imaging pipeline a similar approach is conceivable. After co-registration of histology and MRI volume a new correspondence of MRI slices and new generated histology slices is observable. A registration of these corresponding slices separately in order to correct distortions more accurately could lead to a higher quality of the 3-dimensional histology reconstruction and co-registration of histology and MRI.

A possible problem for the realisation of this approach could be the big difference in the resolution of the the two image modalities. However, no further investigations were made until the release of this thesis.

4.2.3 Non-rigid Registration

The proposed co-registration is adapting an affine transformation in order to align the histology image data to the MRI. The assumption is that even if MRI and histology show structural abnormality in different ways because of different contrast, stains, and characteristics of the image modalities there are enough global shape features that lead to an accurate registration.

In order to provide a more detailed alignment of histology and MRI it is conceivable to use a transformation that allows localised stretching of the images [55 and 56]. A non-rigid transformation would not confine the registration to global transformations like translation, rotation, scaling, and shearing but would enable a local manipulation of voxels.

Unfortunately, it is very difficult to distinguish between anatomical changes and local distortions in histology. A non-rigid registration will likely overfit the histology to the MRI volume which makes further refinement of the correspondences between the two image modalities unlikely. However, no further investigation on these issues were made within the context of this thesis.

4.3 Future Work

Some points which could potentially improve the proposed imaging pipeline have been pointed out. In future it is also possible to enhance the current work with additional features like a microstructural atlas.

Atlases play an important role in the treatment of Alzheimer's [57] and other neuronal diseases. Especially for the navigation in deep brain stimulation is the use of a detailed atlas essential [58–60]. Such studies often consist of a large number of data sets. A detailed segmentation of anatomical structures is therefore extremely time consuming. Atlas based registration allows the combination of information from a group of subjects to analyse them in the standard space of the atlas [22 and 61]. This makes it possible to apply the information of an atlas to different data sets and allow a succinctly summarisation of anatomical variations in a population [47].

However, the quality of a multimodal atlas for MRI and histology that shows microstructural features depends strongly on the quality of the co-registration. The proposed imaging pipeline provides an alignment of histology and MRI with an accuracy of a pixel edge length in the MRI. This allows the study of subtle MRI appearances of structures which are heavily partial-volumed. The generation of a carefully constructed atlas in combination with the proposed imaging pipeline could aid to the understanding of neuronal processes and lead to a more accurate diagnosis of pathological conditions, as well as a more precise treatment.

5
Conclusion

A direct comparison of MR and histological image data leads to a better understanding of the central nervous system. The present thesis describes a methodology that allows the fusion of 2-dimensional fluorescent histology sections of different stains with a corresponding T2- weighted MRI volume. The proposed imaging pipeline consists of a twofold approach which includes the 3-dimensional reconstruction of the histology volume and its co-registration with a MRI volume. The main challenge of the study is the combination of image data from different image modalities that were acquired at different time points. Matters were complicated further by distortions and deformations of the histology sections.

The here presented image pipeline is able to cope with these difficulties by performing an accurate 3-dimensional reconstruction of the histology volume followed by a co-registration that consists of an initial rigid registration and a final affine registration. The intensity based method performs highly consistent over a group of animals and enables a precise overlay of histology and MRI data in the MRI volume space.

The accuracy of the overall registration is assessed by measuring the discrepancy between the position of anatomical landmarks that were selected by experts of the King's College London, Department for Neuroscience. Landmarks were chosen in the histology image space and transformed to the MR image space. The distance to the position of corresponding points previously chosen in the MRI space were measured and resulted in an accuracy of 0.249 mm for image data of healthy rat brains. Considering the resolution of the MRI volume with a voxel size of 0.234 mm $\times$ 0.234 mm $\times$ 0.600 mm, an imaging pipeline is presented that accomplishes a sub-voxel accuracy and therefore outperforms comparable studies [15, 18, 19 and 28].

Furthermore, the imaging pipeline was applied to animals that suffered a stroke. Here, the image data is characterised by additional deformations due to pathological structures. However, these local deformations did not affect global alignment and the evaluation showed that the proposed method performs consistent with a mean error of 0.323 mm for image data of animals with abnormal structures.

The evaluation indicates that the proposed imaging pipeline is highly advantageous in the comparison of information gained from MR and histology image data and enables a detailed analysis of microstructural features seen in the histology and superimposed on the MRI.

Acknowledgement

I would like to express my gratitude and appreciation to:

Bill Crum, who gave me the freedom to think for myself and supported me with a lot of expertise every time I was lost—Mike Modo, who always believed in me and pushed me to consistently improve my work—Andreas, welcher mir in allen Situation mit Rat und Tat zur Seite stand—meiner Familie, welche mich in jeder Hinsicht im Laufe meines Studiums unterstützte—Ed, Ivan, Tony, Cheska, Doris and all the other guys from the lab in London, thanks for making it such a hard decision to go back to Germany (and for the time in the pub...god, I miss the Sun and Doves!)—GG, sorry that you got fired—the developer of elastix, who came up with a excellent registration toolkit—Erasmus, for financial support—Jannis, für viele Diskussionen während des Schreibens (die nicht immer fachspezifisch waren) und dafür dass du meine Musik ausgehalten hast (okay, meistens)—Olli, dafür dass ich immer auf dich zählen kann—Caro, dafür dass es dich gibt.

Abbreviations

ASGD	Adaptive Stochastic Gradient Descent
DAPI	4',6-Diamidino-2-Phenylindole
DNA	Deoxyribonucleic Acid
GFAP	Glial Fibrillary Acidic Protein
MCAO	Middle Cerebral Artery Occlusion
MI	Mutual Information
MR	Magnetic Resonance
MRI	Magnetic Resonance Imaging
NMI	Normalised Mutual Information
PBS	Phosphate Buffered Saline
RGB	Red, Green, Blue
SSD	Sum of Squared Differences

References

1. Modo, M., Hopkins, K. and Virley, D. (2003). Transplantation of neural stem cells modulates apolipoprotein E expression in a rat model of stroke. *Experimental Neurology, 183*(2), 320–329.
2. Ashioti, M., Beech, J. S., Lowe, A. S., Hesselink, M. B. and Modo, M. et al. (2007). Multi-modal characterisation of the neocortical clip model of focal cerebral ischaemia by MRI, behaviour and immunohistochemistry. *Brain Research, 1145*, 177–189.
3. Modo, M., Cash, D., Mellodew, K., Williams, S. C. and Fraser, S. E. et al. (2002). Tracking Transplanted Stem Cell Migration Using Bifunctional, Contrast Agent-Enhanced, Magnetic Resonance Imaging. *NeuroImage, 17*(2), 803–811.
4. Crum, W., Griffin, L. and Hill, D. (2003). Zen and the art of medical image registration: correspondence, homology, and quality. *NeuroImage, 20*(3), 1425–1437.
5. Fischer, B. (2008). Ill-posed medicine—an introduction to image registration. *Inverse Problems, 24*(3), 1–19.
6. Hajnal, J., Hill, D. and Hawkes, D. (2001). *Medical image registration.* CRC Press.
7. Park, H., Piert, M., Khan, A., Shah, R. and Hussain, H. et al. (2008). Registration Methodology for Histological Sections and In Vivo Imaging of Human Prostate. *Academic Radiology, 15*(8), 1027–1039.
8. Cifor, A., Pridmore, T. and Pitiot, A. (2009). Smooth 3-D reconstruction for 2-D histological images. *Information Processing in Medical Imaging, 21*, 350–361.
9. Wirtz, S. (2009). *Simultane Homogenisierung und Registrierung von Bildern histologischer Serienschnitte.* PhD thesis, University of Lübeck.

10. Ourselin, S., Roche, A., Subsol, G. and Pennec, X. (2001). Reconstructing a 3D structure from serial histological sections. *Image and Vision Computing, 19*, 25-31.
11. Beare, R., Richards, K., Murphy, S., Petrou, S. and Reutens, D. (2008). An assessment of methods for aligning two-dimensional microscope sections to create image volumes. *Journal of Neuroscience Methods, 170*(2), 332–344.
12. Chakravarty, M., Bedell, B., Zehntner, S., Evans, A. and Collins, D. L. (2008). Three-dimensional reconstruction of serial histological mouse brain sections. *Biomedical Imaging : From Nano to Macro, 2008*, 987–990.
13. Denk, W. and Horstmann, H. (2004). Serial Block-Face Scanning Electron Microscopy to Reconstruct Three-Dimensional Tissue Nanostructure. *PLoS Biology, 2*(11).
14. Mega, M., Chen, S., Thompson, P. and Woods, R. (1997). Mapping histology to metabolism: coregistration of stained whole-brain sections to premortem PET in Alzheimer's disease. *NeuroImage, 5*(2), 147–153.
15. Choe, A. S., Gao, Y., Li, X., Compton, K. B. and Stepniewska, I. et al. (2011). Accuracy of image registration between MRI and light microscopy in the ex vivo brain. *Magnetic Resonance Imaging, 29*(5), 683–692.
16. Schormann, T., von Matthey, M. and Dabringhaus, A. (1993). Alignment of 3-D brain data sets originating from MR and histology. *Bioimaging, 1*(2), 119–128.
17. Jacobs, M., Windham, J. and Soltanian-Zadeh, H. (1999). Registration and warping of magnetic resonance images to histological sections. *Medical Physics, 26*(8), 1568–1578.
18. Li, G., Nikolova, S. and Bartha, R. (2006). Registration of in vivo magnetic resonance T1-weighted brain images to triphenyltetrazolium chloride stained sections in small animals. *Journal of Neuroscience Methods, 156*(1-2), 368–375.
19. Zhan, Y., Ou, Y., Feldman, M., Tomaszeweski, J. and Davatzikos, C. et al. (2007). Registering Histologic and MR Images of Prostate for Image-based Cancer Detection. *Academic Radiology, 14*(11), 1367–1381.
20. Pelizzari, C. A., Chen, G. T., Spelbring, D. R., Weichselbaum, R. R. and Chen, C. T. (1989). Accurate three-dimensional registration of CT, PET, and/or MR images of the brain. *Journal of Computer Assisted Tomography, 13*(1), 20–26.
21. Xiao, G., Bloch, B. N., Chappelow, J., Genega, E. M. and Rofsky, N. M. et al. (2011). Determining histology-MRI slice correspondences for defining MRI-based disease signatures of prostate cancer. *Computerized Medical Imaging and Graphics, 35*(7-8), 568–78.
22. Ourselin, S., Bardinet, E. and Dormont, D. (2001). Fusion of histological sections and MR images: towards the construction of an atlas of the human basal ganglia. *Medical Image Computing and Computer Assisted Intervention, 2208*, 743–751.

23. Schmitt, O., Modersitzki, J., Heldmann, S., Wirtz, S. and Fischer, B. (2006). Image Registration of Sectioned Brains. *International Journal of Computer Vision, 73*(1), 5–39.
24. Malandain, G., Bardinet, E., Nelissen, K. and Vanduffel, W. (2004). Fusion of autoradiographs with an MR volume using 2-D and 3-D linear transformations. *NeuroImage, 23*(1), 111–127.
25. Hess, A. (1998). A new method for reliable and efficient reconstruction of 3-dimensional images from autoradiographs of brain sections. *Journal of Neuroscience Methods, 84*(1–2), 77–86.
26. Crum, W. R., Camara, O. and Hill, D. L. G. (2006). Generalized overlap measures for evaluation and validation in medical image analysis. *IEEE Transactions on Medical Imaging, 25*(11), 1451–1461.
27. Palm, C., Vieten, A., Salber, D. and Pietrzyk, U. (2009). Evaluation of registration strategies for multi-modality images of rat brain slices. *Physics in Medicine and Biology, 54*(10), 3269–3289.
28. Breen, M. S., Lazebnik, R. S. and Wilson, D. L. (2005). Three-Dimensional Registration of Magnetic Resonance Image Data to Histological Sections with Model-Based Evaluation. *Annals of Biomedical Engineering, 33*(8), 1100–1112.
29. Klein, S., Staring, M., Murphy, K., Viergever, M. and Pluim, J. (2010). Elastix: a toolbox for intensity-based medical image registration. *IEEE Transactions on Medical Imaging, 29*(1), 196–205.
30. Roger, V., Go, A., Lloyd-Jones, D. and Adams, R. (2011). Heart Disease and Stroke Statistics—2011 Update. *Circulation, Journal of the American Heart Association.*
31. Modo, M., Stroemer, R. P., Tang, E., Veizovic, T. and Sowniski, P. et al. (2000). Neurological sequelae and long-term behavioural assessment of rats with transient middle cerebral artery occlusion. *Journal of Neuroscience Methods, 104*(1), 99–109.
32. Dougherty, E. (1992). *Mathematical morphology in image processing.* CRC Press.
33. Tang, S. and Jiang, T. (2004). Nonrigid registration of medical image by linear singular blending techniques. *Pattern Recognition Letters, 25*(4), 399–406.
34. Klein, S., Pluim, J. P. W., Staring, M. and Viergever, M. A. (2009). Adaptive Stochastic Gradient Descent Optimisation for Image Registration. *International Journal of Computer Vision, 81*(3), 227–239.
35. Plakhov, A. and Cruz, P. (2005). A stochastic approximation algorithm with multiplicative step size adaptation. *Journal of Mathematical Science, 120*, 965–973.
36. Pluim, J. P. W., Maintz, J. B. A. and Viergever, M. A. (2003). Mutual-information-based registration of medical images: a survey. *IEEE Transactions on Medical Imaging, 22*(8), 986–1004.

37 Woods, R. P., Cherry, S. R. and Mazziotta, J. C. (1992). Rapid Automated Algorithm for Aligning and Reslicing PET Images. *Journal of Computer Assisted Tomography, 16*(4), 620.

38 Woods, R. and Mazziotta, J. (1993). MRI-PET registration with automated algorithm. *Journal of Computer Assisted Tomography, 17*(4), 536–546.

39 Studholme, C. (1999). An overlap invariant entropy measure of 3D medical image alignment. *Pattern Recognition, 32*(1), 71–86.

40 Wang, D. (2005). Geometric distortion in structural magnetic resonance imaging. *Current Medical Imaging Reviews, 1*(1), 49–60.

41 Watson, G. P. C. (2004). *The Rat Brain in Stereotaxic Coordinates*. Academic Press.

42 Simpson, J. E., Ince, P. G., Shaw, P. J., Heath, P. R. and Raman, R. et al. (2011). Microarray analysis of the astrocyte transcriptome in the aging brain: relationship to Alzheimer's pathology and APOE genotype. *Neurobiology of Aging, 32*(10), 1795–1807.

43 McGeer, P., Akiyama, H. and Itagaki, S. (1989). Immune system response in Alzheimer's disease. *The Canadian Journal of Neurological Science, 16*(4), 516–27.

44 Wu, D. C., Jackson-Lewis, V., Vila, M., Tieu, K. and Teismann, P. et al. (2002). Blockade of microglial activation is neuroprotective in the 1-methyl-4-phenyl-1, 2, 3, 6-tetrahydropyridine mouse model of Parkinson disease. *The Journal of Neuroscience, 22*(5), 1763–1771.

45 Lee, M. K., Stirling, W., Xu, Y., Xu, X. and Qui, D. et al. (2002). Human alpha-synuclein-harboring familial Parkinson's disease-linked Ala-53 –> Thr mutation causes neurodegenerative disease with alpha-synuclein aggregation in transgenic mice. *Proceedings of the National Academy of Sciences of the United States of America, 99*(13), 8968–8973.

46 Modo, M., Mellodew, K., Cash, D. and Fraser, S. (2004). Mapping transplanted stem cell migration after a stroke: a serial, in vivo magnetic resonance imaging study. *NeuroImage, 21*(1), 311–317.

47 Johnson, G. A., Badea, A., Brandenburg, J., Cofer, G. and Fubara, B. et al. (2010). Waxholm space: an image-based reference for coordinating mouse brain research. *NeuroImage, 53*(2), 365–372.

48 Cuadra, M. B., Pollo, C., Bardera, A., Cuisenaire, O. and Villemure, J.-G. et al. (2004). Atlas-based segmentation of pathological MR brain images using a model of lesion growth. *IEEE Transactions on Medical Imaging, 23*(10), 1301–1314.

49 Schubert, N., Pietrzyk, U., Reiel, M. and Palm, C. (2009). Reduktion von Rissartefakten durch nicht-lineare Registrierung in histologischen Schnittbildern. *Bildverarbeitung für die Medizin 2009, 446*, 410–414.

50 Ogier, A. and Dorval, T. (2007). Biased image correction based on empirical mode decomposition. *Image Processing, 1*, 533–536.

51 Dauguet, J., Mangin, J., Delzescaux, T. and Frouin, V. (2004). Robust inter-slice intensity normalization using histogram scale-space analysis. *Medical Image Computing and Computer Assisted Intervention, 3216*, 242–249.

52 Malandain (2003). Intensity Compensation within Series of Images. *Medical Image Computing and Computer Assisted Intervention, 2879*, 41–49.

53 Leong, F. and Brady, M. (2003). Correction of uneven illumination (vignetting) in digital microscopy images. *Journal of Clinical Pathology, 56*(8), 619–621.

54 Likar, B., Maintz, J., Viergever, M. and Pernusï, F. (2000). Retrospective shading correction based on entropy minimization. *Journal of Microscopy, 197*(3), 285–295.

55 Crum, W. R., Hartkens, T. and Hill, D. L. G. (2003). Non-rigid image registration: theory and practice. *The British Journal of Radiology, 77*(2), 140–153.

56 Modersitzki, J. (2009). *FAIR: flexible algorithms for image registration*. Society for Industrial and Applied Mathematics.

57 Thompson, P. M., Mega, M. S., Woods, R. P., Zoumalan, C. I. and Lindshield, C. J. et al. (2001). Cortical change in Alzheimer's disease detected with a disease-specific population-based brain atlas. *Cerebral Cortex, 11*(1), 1–16.

58 Castro, F., Pollo, C., Meuli, R., Maeder, P. and Cuisenaire, O. et al. (2006). A Cross Validation Study of Deep Brain Stimulation Targeting: From Experts to Atlas-Based, Segmentation-Based and Automatic Registration Algorithms. *IEEE Transactions on Medical Imaging, 25*(11), 1440–1450.

59 Krause, M., Fogel, W., Heck, A. and Hacke, W. (2001). Deep brain stimulation for the treatment of Parkinson's disease: subthalamic nucleus versus globus pallidus internus. *Journal of Neurology, 70*(4), 464–470.

60 Benabid, A. (2003). Deep brain stimulation for Parkinson's disease. *Current Opinion in Neurobiology, 13*(6), 696–706.

61 van der Lijn, F., de Bruijne, M., Hoogendam, Y., Klein, S. and Hameeteman, R. et al. (2009). Cerebellum segmentation in MRI using atlas registration and local multi-scale image descriptors. *Biomedical Imaging: From Nano to Macro, 2009*, 221–224.

UNIVERSITÄT ZU LÜBECK

Im Focus das Leben

- Humanmedizin
- Biomedical Engineering
- Entrepreneurship in Digitalen Technologien
- Infection Biology
- Informatik
- Mathematik in Medizin und Lebenswissenschaften
- Medieninformatik
- Medizinische Informatik
- Medizinische Ingenieurwissenschaft
- Molecular Life Science
- Pflege
- Psychologie

www.uni-luebeck.de

Infinite Science Publishing provides a publication platform for excellent theses as well as scientific monographies and conference proceedings for reasonable costs.

These publications enable scientists and research organizations to reach the maximum attention for their results.

The service of Infinite Science Publishing comprises the entire range from the publication of print-ready documents up to cover design as well as copy-editing of single articles.

Infinite Science Publishing is an imprint of the Infinite Science GmbH, a University of Lübeck spin-off and service partner of the BioMedTec Science Campus.

www.infinite-science.de/publishing

Infinite Science GmbH
MFC 1 | BioMedTec Wissenschaftscampus
Maria-Goeppert-Str. 1, 23562 Lübeck
book@infinite-science.de

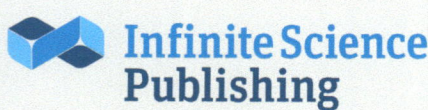